BOVINE RESPIRATORY DISEASE

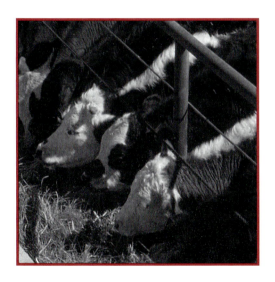

SOURCEBOOK
FOR THE
VETERINARY
PROFESSIONAL

Made possible by an educational grant from

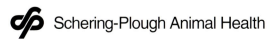

Schering-Plough Animal Health

Library of Congress Card Number: 95-62213

ISBN 1-884254-27-6

Cover illustration: © Grant Heilman, Grant Heilman Photography.

Designed and produced by Veterinary Learning Systems.

Contents

Introduction

Robert A. Smith, DVM, MS, McCasland Chair in
Beef Health and Production
Diplomate ABVP
Boren Veterinary Medical Teaching Hospital
Oklahoma State University
Stillwater, Oklahoma

Bovine respiratory disease (BRD) continues to be a major challenge for the beef industry. In a recent survey, respiratory disease was reported to cause 31.1% of cattle/calf deaths and its economic impact amounted to $624 million.[1] Losses due to death, medical treatment costs, labor, and decreased animal performance affect the economic health of farms, ranches, and feedlots.

Recently weaned beef calves and stocker calves generally experience greater morbidity and mortality rates due to BRD than do yearlings. Often the younger calves have not been immunized and are marketed in smaller groups. BRD is by far the most serious disease entity in this class and age of beef calves. Respiratory disease was responsible for 88.8% of the deaths in Southeastern U.S. beef calves that were shipped to an Oklahoma backgrounding facility between 1983 to 1989.[2] Morbidity rates of stocker calves often exceed 50%. In feedlot cattle, respiratory disease accounts for 65% to 79% of the morbidity[3] and 44% to 72% of the mortality.[3,4] In contrast, death loss due to digestive disorders accounts for 26% of feedlot mortality.

Mortality losses, although more visible, are exceeded by losses in production. In the first 30 days following arrival, calves that remain healthy gain 0.3 to 0.5 lb per day more than calves with BRD.[2,5] One study showed that calves that experienced BRD early in the feeding period gain 0.14 lb less per day during the entire feeding period compared to pen-mates that remained healthy.[3]

Labor costs incurred while caring for sick calves are difficult to calculate due to the multitude of responsibilities assigned to feedlot employees. It is obvious, however, that labor costs are significant.

Proper and efficient management of respiratory disease of stocker and feeder cattle requires a thorough understanding of the etiology, pathogenesis, immunology, epidemiology, clinical signs, therapeutic management, and pathology of the disease complex. It is also vital to understand the interactions that exist among the environment, nutrition, disease agents, and management.

This publication should serve as a detailed, up-to-date reference for bovine practitioners and veterinary students. Bovine respiratory disease is multifactorial; therefore efforts have been made to link the impact of etiologic agents, nutrition, environment, and cattle management with disease incidence.

REFERENCES

1. *Cattle and Calves Death Loss.* National Agricultural Statistics Services, USDA, May 1992.
2. Smith RA, Gill DR: Unpublished data, Pawhuska (Oklahoma) Research Station, 1989.
3. Vogel GJ, Parrott C: Mortality survey in feedyards: The incidence of death from digestive, respiratory, and other causes in feedyards on the Great Plains. *Comp Contin Educ Pract Vet* 16:227–234, 1994.
4. Edwards AJ: The effect of stressors like rumen overload and induced abortion on BRD in feedlot cattle. *Agri-Practice* 10:10–15, 1989.
5. Bateman KG, Martin SW, Shewen PE, Menzies PI: An evaluation of antimicrobial therapy for undifferentiated bovine respiratory disease. *Can Vet J* 31:689–696, 1990.

Etiology, Pathogenesis, and Clinical Signs of Bovine Respiratory Disease

Dee Griffin, DVM, MS, Feedlot Management Specialist
Great Plains Veterinary Education Center
University of Nebraska
Clay Center, Nebraska

ETIOLOGY

Over the past decade, a number of viruses and bacteria/mycoplasma have been associated with acute bovine respiratory disease (BRD).[1] Individually, these pathogens do not appear to be capable of causing disease in healthy cattle.[2] Interactions among many of the bovine respiratory pathogens have been described. Additionally, compromise of the innate respiratory defense mechanisms (in particular, as a result of environmental and management stressors) seems to be critical to the development of clinical BRD.[1,2]

Viruses commonly associated with BRD include[3,4]:

- Bovine herpesvirus 1 (BHV-1) and 3
- Bovine parainfluenza 3 virus (PI_3)
- Bovine viral diarrhea virus (BVDV)
- Bovine respiratory syncytial virus (BRSV)
- Bovine adenovirus
- Bovine rhinovirus
- Bovine reovirus
- Bovine enterovirus
- Bovine coronavirus

BHV-1, PI_3, BVDV, and BRSV are the only viruses that can cause acute respiratory disease without significant interaction with other pathogens.[4] Although BHV-1 is associated with several disease syndromes, it is most often considered a respiratory pathogen. PI_3 is generally a severe respiratory pathogen in young cattle only.[3–5] However, variation in virulence has been noted between strains of this RNA virus. Cases of severe primary disease attributable to PI_3 have been reported in yearling cattle. BRSV is a severe primary respiratory pathogen of newly weaned cattle. BRSV outbreaks in yearling cattle are rare but have been reported.

BVDV is not considered to be a primary respiratory pathogen.[2] Nevertheless, the immunosuppressive nature of this RNA virus is believed to be an important factor in the development of respiratory disease in cattle.[3] Of the other viruses listed above, only adenovirus and rhinovirus have been consistently associated with typical BRD.[2]

In general, bacteria do not serve as primary pathogens of BRD in healthy, unstressed cattle.[4,6] The bacteria and bacteria-like agents that have been most commonly associated with this disease complex include[4,6]:

- *Pasteurella haemolytica*
- *Pasteurella multocida*
- *Haemophilus somnus*
- *Mycoplasma* spp.
- *Chlamydia* spp.

In the High Plains and Midwest United States, *P. haemolytica* type A1 is the most commonly isolated bacterium in fatal cases of BRD.[7] *P. multocida* is believed to cause less fulminating respiratory disease but is reported more often than *P. haemolytica*. *P. multocida* is more commonly isolated in fatal cases of BRD in younger cattle than in fatal cases of BRD in yearling cattle.[8] Because some segments of the cattle feeding industry are handling younger cattle, this pathogen may become increasingly important.

H. somnus has not been reported as commonly in fatal cases of BRD in the High Plains and Midwest as it has been in Canada.[3,5,a] This observation has created controversy about the role of *H. somnus* in BRD in moderate climates. Discrepancies in isolation rates of fatal cases of BRD may not be associated with climatic differences. Differences in livestock genetics and production practices among regions may be associated with the reported isolations of the organism.

Mycoplasma and *Chlamydia* spp. are commonly isolated by some diagnostic laboratories. Neither is considered a primary pathogen in weaned or yearling cattle. These organisms are often isolated in association with other respiratory bacterial pathogens, and their role in BRD apparently involves their interaction with these other pathogens.[2]

The etiology of BRD cases identified late in the feeding period can be difficult to determine. The highest incidence occurs in the spring as ambient temperatures begin to approach the upper critical temperature for cattle (60° to 65° F). Previous pneumonia is a common postmortem finding. Attempts to link these cases to a particular viral, bacterial, fungal, or chemical agent have been unrewarding.

Environmental, nutritional, and management stressors are not primary etiologic agents. The role of these stressors in the onset of clinical BRD is discussed later.

The relationship between genetics and BRD is unclear. Genetic mapping is presently underway at several research stations across the United States. Recent work at the Roman L. Hruska U.S. Meat Animal Research Center suggests that a relationship may exist between genetics and BRD.[9]

PATHOGENESIS

The pathogenesis of viral agents of BRD is usually related to the cellular damage caused by their local replication. Lysis of cells and the release of cellular debris act as mediators of inflammation.[5,9,10] It is believed that respiratory viruses compromise respiratory defense mechanisms to allow bacterial pathogens access to the lower respiratory tract. The relationship of these two events has not been consistently associated with the onset of clinical BRD.[10,11] Environmental and management stressors are a third factor commonly associated with the development of clinical BRD.[10,12]

The damage to the upper respiratory tract caused by the respiratory viruses allows potential bacterial pathogens access to the lung. Viral replication in the ciliated epithelium results in a loss of this important pulmonary clearance mechanism. Damage is not limited to the ciliated epithelium. Viral replication and subsequent damage along the entire mucosal surface further disarm the immune system by eliminating the capability for local antibody production and providing suitable sites for bacterial replication. While BHV-1 is noted for its severe upper respiratory tract damage, PI_3 and BRSV also share this capability.[13–15]

Viral damage is not limited to the upper respiratory tract. The respiratory viruses compromise the cellular function and architecture of the terminal bronchi and alveolar wall.[13–15] Inflammation of these structures leads to plugging of the airways and is in part responsible for the soft, nonproductive cough that usually develops. In some cases movement of the virus from the alveolar wall to the interstitium results in interstitial edema and emphysema.

Environmental stresses include heat or cold stress, respirable dust, and fumes toxic to the respiratory epithelium. Management stresses that lead to dehydration and increased levels of circulating glucocorticoids play an important role in disarming an animal's respiratory defense mechanisms.[1,2] Once the innate defense mechanisms are disarmed, potential bacterial pathogens that normally reside in the upper respiratory tract are allowed access to the lung.[3,12,16] An aerosol of *P. haemolytica* has

---

[a]See article on p. 12.

been shown to make cattle susceptible to BHV-1.[14] Therefore it should not be supposed that the bacterial component of BRD necessarily follows a viral infection. However, viral vaccination has been shown to be protective against experimentally induced *P. haemolytica* challenge.[1,2]

P. haemolytica type A1 is found in the upper respiratory tract of sick cattle more often than any of the other 15 serotypes of this species. Although aerosol infection has been produced with this bacterium, the communicability of this serotype is not well characterized.[17]

P. haemolytica type A1 causes the most severe damage of all of the recognized bacterial pathogens.[14,18] The presence of this organism is associated with coagulative necrosis, fibrin, and edema. Lesions of this type suggest severe vascular damage.[14] The functional destruction of pulmonary tissue can be extensive. *P. haemolytica* produces a potent cytotoxic exotoxin and leukotoxin. The production of exotoxin peaks within 6 hours of infection. The leukotoxin produced destroys the alveolar macrophages and the neutrophils that accumulate in response to the infection. The resulting release of proteolytic enzymes and oxidants damages cellular membranes and increases capillary permeability. Fluid accumulates in the interstitium of the alveolar wall, causing alveolar necrosis and pulmonary edema.[14]

P. multocida causes less damage in the respiratory tract than does *P. haemolytica*.[14] However, its frequency of isolation from fatal cases of BRD in cattle less than 7 months of age makes it a primary concern in many operations. *P. multocida, Fusobacterium necrophorum,* and *Actinomyces pyogenes* are consistently isolated from laryngeal abscesses from cattle in the Southern Plains states suffering from the so-called "hard breather" syndrome. Affected cattle have typically been on feed for several months. The role of viruses in this syndrome is unclear.

In the High Plains and Midwest United States the role of other bacterial agents in the pathogenesis of BRD is not well defined. *H. somnus* is believed to cause septicemia with localization in the lung and other tissues. The fact that *H. somnus* is a facultative intracellular organism makes it more difficult for the host to defend itself. Adhesion along the vascular endothelium causes vasculitis with subsequent desquamation and exposure of the subendothelial layer and leads to thrombosis. Ischemic necrosis of adjacent parenchyma and extensive fibrin production are common sequelae. Multiple body systems are often involved. *Mycoplasma* and *Chlamydia* spp. may share a similar mechanism.[2]

Some cattle with fatal cases of BRD seem to have only minimal lung damage.[4,14] This suggests the mechanism involved in fatal cases is more complex than can be explained by loss of pulmonary function. The role of the mediators of inflammation is discussed later.

The role of nutritional components in the pathogenesis of BRD has been a subject of controversy. Several studies have investigated the relationship between BRD and micronutrients. Copper and vitamin E have been the most common micronutrients evaluated. Few studies have shown a relationship between micronutrient supplementation and clinical BRD. The mechanisms of the micronutrients' protective effects with respect to BRD are thought to relate to immune cellular function.[2,5,6] It is important to note that not all studies have shown similar results.

CLINICAL SIGNS

Clinical signs of BRD usually develop 5 to 14 days following environmental or management stresses. Variation in the clinical signs of BRD is associated with the multitude of etiologic factors involved in the disease process. Signs include anorexia, rapid respiration, generalized depression and weakness, coughing, increased nasal and ocular discharge, and high body temperatures (Table 1). The onset can be very dramatic, with some cattle found dead and a large percentage in a group showing severe depression.[1,9,14]

TABLE 1
Signs Associated with BRD

Anorexia

Depression

Increased breathing rate

Soft coughing

Nasal discharge

Watery eyes

Abnormal abdominal fill

Stiff movement

Loose feces

Elevated body temperature

Because treatment early in the disease process is considered important, a detailed list of signs is presented. Many of the signs discussed are not specific to BRD but are useful considerations when attempting to identify affected cattle early in the disease process. It is important to note that packing house surveys have not consistently shown a relationship between pulmonary scars and identification of previous respiratory disease.

In experimentally induced BRD the most common and perhaps most important early sign is appetite depression. Decreased feed intake has been documented to occur 24 to 48 hours prior to an increase in body temperature.[4] Excellent feed intake records can provide important information for detecting BRD early in the disease process in individual groups of cattle. This information is less valuable in groups that have been mixed together and in which disease may not be in the same stage of incubation. Decreased feed intake in a group of cattle can signal the need for closer observation of individual animals. Changes in individual cattle feed intake can be evaluated by carefully observing the shape of the animal's abdomen. A slight abdominal bounce can often be observed in sick cattle. Cattle that have been anorexic for more than 24 hours exhibit an abdominal tuck or slab-sided appearance. Any deviation in the character of the feces should be considered important. Diarrhea is more common than firm stools in cattle suffering from BRD.

The respiratory rate in cattle can be very difficult to evaluate. Fermentation of feed in the rumen and ambient temperatures that approach the upper critical temperature (60° to 65° F) compound the difficulty of using respiratory rates as a useful clinical observation.[19] For respiratory rate to be useful, cattle must be examined before the ambient temperature reaches upper critical temperature and before feed fermentation in the rumen has had time to alter the respiratory rate. For this reason, it is much more difficult to evaluate cattle observed or treated in the afternoon.

In the early stages of BRD a slight, generalized depression can be noticed. Cattle hold their head slightly lower than normal. Those suffering from an emphysematous reaction typically elevate their head. Their attitude is a bit distant, and they are less interested in what is occurring in their environment. Their hair grooming habits are not as vigorous as those of normal cattle. Often affected cattle appear to be trying to hide behind other cattle, between cattle eating at the feed bunk, or in the corner of the pen near the end of the feed bunk. To notice slight changes in depression, it is important to move all cattle and get a good look at each animal.

Cattle with BRD often have slightly stiffer movements than normal and exhibit a shortened stride. Affected animals may drag their toes or knuckle slightly. Their tail may appear to be tucked slightly between their hocks. Depression and dehydration become more pronounced as BRD progresses.

The cough associated with BRD is usually soft and repetitive. Early in the disease, cattle suffering from BRD often have watery, dull eyes and a clear nasal discharge. It may be observed that they rapidly lick their nostrils yet have a relatively dirty nose. The sclera, third eyelid, and visible mucous membranes inside the nostrils often appear reddened. As BRD progresses, the nose often becomes crusty and tear staining can be noticed.

Cattle that develop BRD late in the feeding period typically develop severe dyspnea. Many have an elevated head, excessive salivation, and an expiratory press. Their attitude is anxious and belligerent because of their severe anoxia. These cases are usually diagnosed as atypical interstitial pneumonia (AIP) and are often blamed on BRSV; it is not unusual for laboratory samples to be fluorescent antibody positive for BRSV. I believe many of these cases are associated with unresolved bacterial infections during times of mild heat stress.

In the Southern Plains states, two additional respiratory syndromes—the hard breather and honker syndromes—may be seen in the late feeding period. Unlike the emphysematous reaction often found in late feeding period BRD, these syndromes (both are upper respiratory diseases) often involve a similar respiratory honking sound. Affected cattle also appear anxious and belligerent. An expiratory press is typically absent. Both conditions are life-threatening emergencies.

The temperature of cattle suffering from BRD ranges from 103° to 108° F. Variation in individual animals is influenced by the stage of disease, ambient temperature, design of examination/treatment facilities, temperament of the animal, and the animal handling ability of the people caring for sick cattle.

High body temperatures in cattle that appear relatively bright and alert are most often observed in the early stages of disease. As the disease progresses, high body temperature in severely depressed animals is often a grave sign.

REFERENCES

1. Smith RA: A review of bovine respiratory disease. *Bovine Proc* 16:102–121, 1984.
2. Thomson RG: The pathogenesis and lesions of pneumonia in cattle. *Compend Contin Educ Pract Vet* 3(11):S403–S411, 1981.
3. Pringle JK, Viel L, Shewen PE, et al: Bronchoalveolar lavage of cranial and caudal lung regions in selected normal calves: Cellular, microbiological, immunoglobulin, serological and histological variables. *Can J Vet Res* 52:239–248, 1988.
4. Yates WDG, Kingscote BF, Bradley JA, Mitchell D: The relationship of serology and nasal microbiology to pulmonary lesions in feedlot cattle. *Can J Comp Med* 47:375–378, 1983.
5. Ryan AM, Hutcheson DP, Womack JE: Type-I interferon genotypes and severity of clinical disease in cattle inoculated with bovine herpesvirus 1. *Am J Vet Res* 54(1):73–79, 1993.
6. Magwood SE, Barnum DA, Thomson RG: Nasal bacterial flora of calves in healthy and in pneumonia-prone herds. *Can J Comp Med* 33:237–243, 1969.
7. Binkhorst GJ, Henricks PAJ, v d Ingh TSGAM, et al: The effect of stress on host defense system and on lung damage in calves experimentally infected with *Pasteurella haemolytica* type A 1. *J Vet Med A* 37:525– 536, 1990.
8. Griffin DD: Managing the health problems in feedlots. *DVM Magazine* 24(8):6a–10a, 1993.
9. Muggli-Cockett NE, Cundiff LV, Gregory KE: Genetic analysis of bovine respiratory disease in beef calves during the first year of life. *J Anim Sci* 70:2013–2019, 1992.
10. Frank GH: The role of *Pasteurella haemolytica* in the bovine respiratory disease complex. *Vet Med Food Anim Pract* 838–846, 1986.
11. Frank GH, Briggs RE: Colonization of the tonsils of calves with *Pasteurella haemolytica*. *Am J Vet Res* 53(4):481–484, 1992.
12. Frank GH, Smith PC: Prevalence of *Pasteurella haemolytica* in transported calves. *Am J Vet Res* 44(6):981–985, 1983.
13. Briggs RE, Frank GH: Increased elastase activity in nasal mucus associated with nasal colonization by *Pasteurella haemolytica* in infectious bovine rhinotracheitis virus-infected calves. *Am J Vet Res* 53(5):631–635, 1992.
14. Daoust PY: Morphological study of bacterial pneumonia of feedlot cattle: Determination of age of lesions. *Can Vet J* 30:155–160, 1989.
15. Engen RL, Brown TT Jr: Changes in phospholipids of alveolar lining material in calves after aerosol exposure to bovine herpesvirus-1 or parainfluenza-3 virus. *Am J Vet Res* 52(5): 675–677, 1991.
16. Weiss DJ, Bauer MC, Whiteley LO, et al: Changes in blood and bronchoalveolar lavage fluid components in calves with experimentally induced pneumonic pasteurellosis. *Am J Vet Res* 52(2):337–344, 1991.
17. Martin SW, Darlington G, Bateman K, Holt J: Undifferentiated bovine respiratory disease (shipping fever): Is it communicable? *Prev Vet*

Med 6:27–35, 1988.

18. Simons KR, Morton RJ, Fulton RW, Confer AW: Comparison of antibody responses in cattle to outer membrane proteins from *Pasteurella haemolytica* serotype 1 and from eight untypeable strains. *Am J Vet Res* 53(6):971–975, 1992.

19. Hahn GL: Body temperature rhythms in farm animals—A review and reassessment relative to environmental influences. Proceedings of the 11th ISB-Congress, West Lafayette, 1989, pp 325–337.

Haemophilus somnus: An Important Feedlot Pathogen

P.T. Guichon, DVM
G.K. Jim, DVM
C.W. Booker, DVM, MVetSc
O.C. Schunicht, DVM, BSc
Feedlot Health Management Services
Okotoks, Alberta, Canada

Haemophilus somnus infection (or hemophilosis) is becoming increasingly recognized as the primary cause of death in calves in western Canadian feedlots.[1-3] *H. somnus* was first identified in cattle in 1956. At that time thromboembolic meningoencephalitis (TME) appeared to be the only clinical manifestation of *H. somnus* infection. Although TME is still seen today, its incidence appears to be decreasing.[1] It is now known that *H. somnus* causes disease in both the upper (Figure 1) and lower respiratory tract (Figure 2).[1]

EPIDEMIOLOGY

H. somnus is a gram-negative bacterium that is not capable of surviving for long periods outside the host organism under most circumstances. However, it can survive up to 75 days in biologic secretions, which may allow it to overwinter.[4] It also survives in urine for short periods, which may be an important feature in animal to animal transmission in confined feedlot cat-

tle. Animal to animal transmission may also occur when animals inhale aerosolized bacterial particles. *H. somnus* resides in the reproductive tract of both males and females, and it is likely that this is the reservoir of the organism.[1,5,6]

Serologic evidence suggests that calves placed in the feedlot are exposed to both *Pasteurella haemolytica* and *H. somnus* in the early feeding period.[7] Van Donkersgoed and associates reported that *H. somnus* titers increased significantly ($P < 0.05$) in unvaccinated calves from feedlot entry to day 96 of the feeding period.[8] They also reported that calves that experienced two relapses of BRD or died as a result of BRD or hemophilosis had lower *H. somnus* titers than did animals in which relapse or death did not occur. According to Guichon and coworkers, titers to *P. haemolytica* and *H. somnus* increased sharply in calves 18 days after feedlot arrival, suggesting that animals were exposed to both pathogens.[7] In addition, they concluded that animals with lower *H. som-*

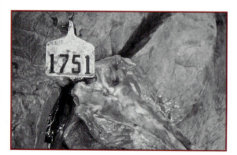

Figure 1. Laryngitis due to *H. somnus*.

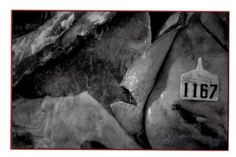

Figure 2. Bronchopneumonia due to *H. somnus*.

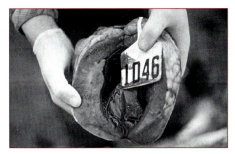

Figure 3. Myocardial lesion caused by *H. somnus* infection.

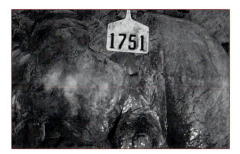

Figure 4. Pulmonary edema.

nus titers at feedlot arrival were at greater risk of dying than were animals with higher titers. Further, cattle that developed fever in the first month of the feeding period had higher mortality as a result of hemophilosis as well as higher overall mortality than did cattle that did not develop fever. Undifferentiated fever was a useful criterion for identifying cattle that required therapy, as animals that developed fever were five times more likely to die of all causes and ten times more likely to die of hemophilosis than were animals that did not develop fever.

Orr reported a seasonal increase in the number of cases of *H. somnus* submitted to a veterinary diagnostic laboratory at the University of Saskatchewan.[9] Most necropsies were received at the laboratory during the months of November, December, and January. Orr concluded that over a 20 year period there was an "increased importance of respiratory and myocardial diseases caused by this organism."

Epidemiologic data collected on feedlot calves in western Canada indicate that animals suffering fatal fibrinous pneumonia are first treated after less than 14 days on feed. In contrast, animals suffering fatal hemophilosis are first treated after they have been on feed for 3 weeks. Similarly, animals suffering fatal fibrinous pneumonia die less than 30 days on feed whereas calves with fatal hemophilosis die within 30 to 60 days on feed. Other retrospective mortality surveys in western Canada report similar findings.[2]

CLINICAL SIGNS

Animals suffering from the various manifestations of hemophilosis present clinically different signs to the veterinarian or the feedlot penchecker. Signs of neurologic dysfunction, including knuckling of the hind limbs, ataxia, opisthotonus, and hyperextension of the neck in recumbent animals, are evidence of TME. While some animals appear moribund, others without any evidence of preexisting clinical disease are found dead in the pen. Animals suffering from myocardial infarction due to *H. somnus* infection may also be discovered dead in the pen, exhibit clinical signs similar to BRD, or show evidence of congestive heart failure. The myocardial lesions typically appear in the myocardium of the left ventricle. The lesion can range from an ovoid necrotic area (Figure 3) to a purulent abscess. Animals suffering pericardial lesions, pneumonia, or pleuritis due to *H. somnus* infection exhibit signs similar to those associated with other forms of BRD. Pulmonary edema often appears secondarily to cardiac lesions (Figure 4). Many animals develop polyarthritis, which is predominantly evident clinically in one or both stifle joints but may occur in other joints as well. In cases of fatal hemophilosis, the history often includes prior treatment for BRD.[2]

Studies have shown that weaned calves inoculated intrabronchially with *H. somnus* developed more severe respiratory disease when previously exposed to bovine respiratory syncytial virus (BRSV) or infectious bovine rhinotracheitis (IBR) virus.[1] In addition to

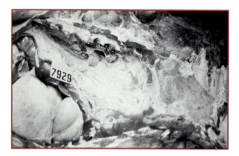

Figure 5. Pleuritis due to *H. somnus* infection.

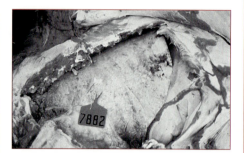

Figure 6. Septicemia due to *H. somnus* infection.

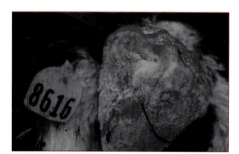

Figure 7. Pericarditis due to *H. somnus* infection.

penumonia, *H. somnus* can cause a severe fibrinous pleuritis[1] (Figure 5), myocarditis[1,10] (Figure 3), septicemia (Figure 6), and pericarditis (Figure 7) and has been implicated in polyarthritis (Figure 8).

As shown in Table 1, myocarditis, pericarditis, pneumonia, pleuritis, TME, and septicemia accounted for 33% of the mortality in western Canadian feedlots. If polyarthritis is included in the hemophilosis category, *H. somnus* infection is potentially implicated in 40% of all mortality in this population. In contrast, less than 30% of the feedlot mortality was due to fibrinous pneumonia or pasteurellosis. If these mortality rates represent morbidity rates within the general feedlot population, BRD is as likely to be caused by *H. somnus* infection as by *Pasteurella*. Retrospective mortality studies indicate that within large calf populations, approximately 1% of the animals will succumb to a form of hemophilosis.[2,8]

DIAGNOSIS

Necropsy diagnosis of hemophilosis in feedlot cattle may be difficult. When necropsies are conducted in the field, an examination of the brain is unlikely unless the animal had neurologic signs prior to death. In cases of TME the hemorrhagic necrosis in the brain may only be recognizable via histopathology and the animal may be misdiagnosed as suffering from another neurologic disease (e.g., polioencephalomalacia). Pulmonary edema associated with cardiac failure due to a myocardial infarct can be misdiagnosed as an interstitial pneumonia (falsely implicating hemophilosis), particularly if the heart is not examined thoroughly. Septicemic feedlot calves often die in the pen without signs of clinical disease prior to death, and blood culture is required to confirm the existence of *H. somnus*. Culturing of *H. somnus* from lung tissue in the laboratory is necessary to confirm a diagnosis of *H. somnus* pneumonia. It should be noted that it may be difficult to culture *H. somnus* if the animal has been treated with antimicrobials and that differences in microbiologic technique may influence the ability of a diagnostic laboratory to culture the organism. It has also been suggested that in some cases to which a diagnosis of pasteurellosis has been ascribed, *H. somnus* may be the primary pathogen.[1] It is speculated that *H. somnus* involvement is overlooked because *P. haemolytica* can overgrow the slower growing *H. somnus* on culture or there may be

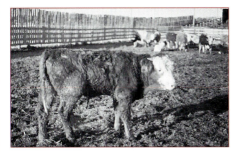
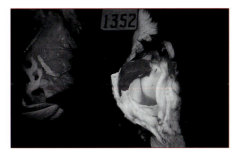

Figure 8A   **Figure 8B**

Figure 8. Polyarthritis due to *H. somnus* infection.

TABLE 1
Specific Cause of Mortality in High Risk, Fall-Placed Feedlot Calves (n = 118,828) in Western Canada (period ending January 31, 1995)

Cause of Death	*Number of Deaths*	*Proportional Mortality*	*Absolute Mortality*
Bloat	228	11.7	0.19
Fibrinous pneumonia	574	29.5	0.48
Haemophilus myocarditis	182	9.4	0.15
Haemophilus pericarditis	46	2.4	0.04
Haemophilus pleuritis	187	9.7	0.16
Haemophilus pneumonia	16	0.8	0.01
Haemophilus septicemia	171	8.8	0.14
Other metabolic causes	30	1.5	0.03
Miscellaneous	236	12.1	0.20
Polyarthritis	141	7.3	0.12
Other respiratory causes	102	5.2	0.09
Thrombotic meningoencephalitis	31	1.6	0.03
TOTAL	1944	100	1.64

differences in the sensitivity of the organisms to previous antimicrobial therapy that may prevent culture of *H. somnus.*

TREATMENT

H. somnus is very sensitive to therapeutic levels of most antimicrobials, including tetracycline, florfenicol, sulfonamides, and cephalosporins. Unfortunately, it is difficult to assess treatment of hemophilosis for several reasons. First, it is not known whether the animal is suffering from *H. somnus* infection at the time it is pulled and treated for undifferentiated fever. Second, many animals are simply found dead in the pen or are given therapy for a short time (less than 2 days) prior to death. Third, respiratory infections are often complicated by pathogens other than *H. somnus,* including *Pasteurella* spp. and viruses, which may influence therapy outcome. As a result of these factors, treatment response rates and case fatality rates associated with administration of various antimicrobials to animals with *H. somnus* infection are unknown.

PREVENTION

Measures to control *H. somnus* infection are less than adequate. Vaccination has been recommended prior to infection, with revaccination 2 to 4 weeks later to maximize the immune response.[11-13] Laboratory studies have shown that vaccination is efficacious in calves challenged with a virulent *H. somnus* strain[11-13] and is effective in reducing disease in field situations.[11,13-18] It has been speculated that *H. somnus* mortality rates are increasing as the result of mass treatment programs, the development of different or more virulent *H. somnus* strains, or the general ability of the organism to adapt.[1] In the feedlot it is logical to assume that calves are exposed to *H. somnus* upon feedlot arrival and that initial infection may occur prior to development of adequate protection as a result of vaccination. In addition, most feedlots lack the enthusiasm to revaccinate cattle 14 to 28 days after feedlot arrival without field evidence of the cost effectiveness of this procedure.

Recent research has concluded that mass feeding of prophylactic antibiotics for extended periods has reduced hemophilosis mortality in the feedlot.[19] Further work is necessary to confirm these observations.

CONCLUSION

H. somnus is a contributor to morbidity and mortality in feedlot calves in the early feeding period. It produces several distinct clinical and pathologic conditions in feedlot calves including TME, myocarditis, pleuritis, pericarditis, pneumonia, septicemia, and polyarthritis. Its exact role in producing undifferentiated fever in calves is not well understood, nor is it clear why animals succumb to any of the particular manifestations of the disease. The organism is often isolated with other known pathogens, and it may act as a primary or secondary pathogen. One should not automatically assume that cattle pulled and treated in the early feeding period have pasteurellosis; rather, they may be suffering from *H. somnus* infection.

REFERENCES

1. Harris FW, Janzen ED: The *Haemophilus somnus* disease complex (hemophilosis): A review. *Can Vet J* 30:816–822, 1989.
2. Van Donkersgoed J, Janzen ED, Harland RJ: Epidemiological features of calf mortality due to hemophilosis in a large feedlot. *Can Vet J* 31:821–825, 1990.
3. Jim GK, Guichon PT, Shaw G: Protecting calves from pneumonic pasteurellosis. *Vet Med* 83:1084–1087, 1988.
4. Dewey KJ, Little PB: Environmental survival of *Haemophilus somnus* and influence of secretions and excretions. *Can J Comp Med* 45:23–26, 1984.
5. Humphrey JD, Little PB, Barnum DA, et al: Occurrence of *Haemophilus somnus* in bovine semen and in the prepuce of bulls and steers. *Can J Comp Med* 46:215–217, 1982.
6. Humphrey JD, Little PB, Stephens LR, et al: Prevalence and distribution of *Haemophilus somnus* in the male bovine reproductive tract. *Am J Vet Res* 43:791–795, 1982.
7. Guichon PT, Harland RJ, Booker CW, Jim GK: Serological differences in feedlot cattle suffering from undifferentiated fever. Farming For The Future Program, Alberta Agriculture Project #920215.
8. Van Donkersgoed J, Janzen ED, Potter AA, Harland RJ: The occurrence of *Haemophilus somnus* in feedlot calves and its control by post arrival prophylactic mass medication. *Can Vet J* 35:573–580, 1994.
9. Orr JP: *Haemophilus somnus* infection: A retrospective analysis of cattle necropsied at the Western College of Veterinary Medicine from 1970 to 1990. *Can Vet J* 33:719–722, 1992.
10. Guichon PT, Pritchard J, Jim GK: *Haemophilus somnus* myocarditis in a feedlot steer. *Can Vet J* 29:1012–1013, 1988.
11. Saunders JR, Janzen ED: *Haemophilus somnus* infections II. A Canadian field trial of a commercial bacterin: Clinical and serological results. *Can Vet J* 21:219–224, 1980.
12. Groom SC, Little PB: Vaccination of cattle against experimentally induced *Haemophilus somnus* pneumonia. *Am J Vet Res* 49:793–800, 1988.
13. Stephens LR, Little PB, Humphrey JD, et al: Vaccination of cattle against experimentally induced thromboembolic meningoencephalitis with a *Haemophilus somnus* bacterin. *Am J Vet Res* 43:1339–1342, 1982.
14. Ribble CS, Jim GK, Janzen ED: Efficacy of immunization of feedlot calves with a commercial *Haemophilus somnus* bacterin. *Can J Vet Res* 52:191–198, 1988.

15. Amstutz HE, Horstman LA, Morter RL: Clinical evaluation of the efficacy of *Haemophilus somnus* and *Pasteurella sp.* bacterins. *Bovine Pract* 16:106–108, 1981.
16. Hall RF, Williams JM, Smith GL: Field evaluation of *Haemophilus somnus* bacterin. *Vet Med Small Anim Clin* 72:1368–1370, 1977.
17. Van Donkersgoed J, Schumann FJ, Harland RJ, et al: The effect of route and dosage of immunization on the serological response to a *Pasteurella haemolytica* and *Haemophilus somnus* vaccine in feedlot calves. *Can Vet J* 34:731–735, 1993.
18. Van Donkersgoed J, Potter AA, Mollison B, Harland RJ: The effect of a combined *Pasteurella haemolytica* and *Haemophilus somnus* vaccine and a modified-live bovine respiratory syncytial virus vaccine against enzootic pneumonia in young beef calves. *Can Vet J* 35:239–241, 1994.
19. Guichon PT, Jim GK, Booker CW: An evaluation of AUREO® S-700 for the reduction of feedlot disease and improvement in feedlot performance, in press.

Immunology and Prevention of Bovine Respiratory Disease

Louis J. Perino, DVM, PhD, Beef Cattle Herd Health
Management Veterinarian and Associate Professor
Great Plains Veterinary Educational Center
University of Nebraska
Clay Center, Nebraska

IMMUNOLOGY OF THE RESPIRATORY TRACT

Most economically significant cattle diseases occur at mucosal surfaces, such as the respiratory tract. Mucosal immunity must overcome the unique challenges at this interface, such as absorption, secretion, and gas exchange. Several complex, interrelated defense mechanisms protect the respiratory system from infectious agents. Such defenses can be either innate (e.g., intact epithelium, mucus, ciliated epithelial cells, complement, interferon, natural killer cells, and phagocytes) or acquired (e.g., antibodies and cytotoxic T lymphocytes).

The upper and lower respiratory tracts are quite different and present different challenges to the immune system. The upper respiratory system is far from sterile. It normally harbors a number of organisms, including *Pasteurella* spp. and *Haemophilus somnus*.[1,2] The main defense systems in this part of the respiratory tract are noninflammatory and are directed toward preventing pathogen adherence. Innate defenses include the production of a layer of mucus and the clearing activity of ciliated epithelium. Together, mucus and ciliated epithelium form the mucociliary escalator, which traps and clears infectious agents from the upper respiratory tract, preventing pathogens from establishing infection. As a result of the action of the mucociliary escalator, as well as that of the turbulence produced by air passing through the upper respiratory tract, all but the smallest particles (<5 microns) are filtered from incoming air. Another important defense mechanism involves the production of interferon by virus-infected cells, which helps protect neighboring cells from virus infection.

Acquired immunity also contributes to the defense of the upper respiratory tract through secretory antibody activity. IgA is the primary antibody involved; IgG may also be important, especially in ruminants.[3] The role of cytotoxic T cells in defending the upper respiratory tract is not as well characterized.

Normally, the lower respiratory tract is a sterile environment. The main defense systems are inflammatory and are directed toward killing and clearing infectious agents. As does the upper respiratory tract, the lower respiratory tract has innate defense mechanisms. Alveolar macrophages form an important first line of such defenses. Once infection occurs, complement and neutrophils make up a second echelon of innate defense. Acquired immune defenses in the form of immunoglobulins and cytotoxic T lymphocytes also contribute to pathogen clearance.

The importance of the innate defenses in both parts of the respiratory tract cannot be overemphasized. In evidence of this, introducing bacteria into the respiratory tract does not induce pneumonia unless the innate defenses are deranged.[4,5]

Host-Pathogen Interactions in Bovine Respiratory Disease

While the calf's respiratory tract arrays many defenses against potential pathogens, the relationship between the calf and the pathogen is dynamic, with microbes employing several strategies to blunt host defenses.[6] These include tolerance, immunosuppression, infection of sites inaccessible to the immune response, ineffective antibody induction, consumption of antibodies by soluble antigens, local interference, antigenic variation, avoidance of induction of an immune response, and reduced induction of or responsiveness to interferon.

One consideration is whether the pathogen has an intracellular or an extracellular life-style. This is particularly relevant in terms of the types of immune effector mechanisms (antibodies or cytotoxic cells) important in fighting infection. Viruses are obligate intracellular pathogens, although they may be exposed to extracellular immune mechanisms during different stages of infection. Other respiratory pathogens have more variable growth requirements. Some, such as *Mycoplasma* spp. and *H. somnus*, are facultative intracellular pathogens. Others, such as *Pasteurella* spp., have a predominantly extracellular life-style.

Primary viral infections may independently cause clinical disease, depending on the type of virus and condition of the host. More importantly, they predispose an animal to secondary complications such as bacterial infection, particularly when other immunosuppressive factors are present. Such factors include stress, poor nutrition, and/or concurrent disease. Viral infections interact in this complex system to induce detrimental effects on host defense mechanisms.

Immunosuppressive effects of some bovine viral pathogens are manifested by their ability to facilitate bacterial colonization of the lower respiratory tract.[4] In several studies, aerosol exposure to bovine herpesvirus 1 (BHV-1) facilitates lung infection by a usually noninfectious dose of *Pasteurella haemolytica,* resulting in fibrinous pneumonia.[2,7–11] In another investigation, after calves cleared *P. haemolytica*

serotype 1 from their nasal passages, intranasal inoculation with BHV-1 caused recrudescence of *P. haemolytica* infection in two of eight calves.[12] Calves recently infected with or seroconverting to bovine viral diarrhea virus (BVDV) have been reported to experience increased incidence of bacterial infection.[13] Under appropriate experimental conditions, BVDV also facilitates pneumonic infection by a usually noninfectious dose of *P. haemolytica*.[14] BVDV infection reportedly predisposes cattle to development of bacterial pneumonia following aerosol exposure to *P. haemolytica*[15–17] or *P. multocida*.[18,19] Bovine respiratory syncytial virus (BRSV) may also predispose cattle to secondary bacterial pneumonia.[20,21]

Specific mechanisms by which viral pathogens affect the immune system include derangement of the mucociliary escalator as well as alteration of bovine alveolar macrophage, neutrophil, and lymphocyte functions.

In vitro and in vivo experiments show cytopathic effects on respiratory epithelium that result in compromised mucociliary defense mechanisms.[22,23] BVDV readily destroys ciliary activity in infected cultures of bovine tracheal rings.[24] Aerosol exposure of calves to parainfluenza-3 virus (PI$_3$) followed by aerosol exposure to *P. haemolytica* results in reduced clearance of *P. haemolytica*.[25–27] Electron microscopy of 1-month-old calves infected with BRSV demonstrates that viral assembly and release in tracheal and bronchial epithelial cells are associated with cilia loss.[28]

The bovine alveolar macrophage is a pivotal cell in the innate defense network of the lung. BHV-1 reportedly has cytopathic effects on bovine alveolar macrophages,[24,29] even though it appears to replicate in bovine alveolar macrophages at very low levels[29–31] or not at all.[24] Other BHV-1–mediated effects noted in these in vitro bovine alveolar macrophage studies include reductions in F$_c$-mediated receptor activity and phagocytosis, complement receptor activity, and antibody-dependent cellular cytotoxicity.[31] In vitro studies on bovine alveolar macrophages indicate BVDV is capable of replicating and causing cytopathic effects.[24,29] Similarly, cytopathic effects are seen in bovine alveolar macrophage cultures infected in vitro with PI$_3$.[24,29] Additionally, infected bovine alveolar macrophages show depressed phagocytic activity against *Candida glabrata* and marked reduction in phagosome/lysosome fusion.[32] In vitro inoculation of bovine alveolar macrophages with BRSV impairs selected functions[33]; F$_c$-mediated phagocytosis of antibody-coated sheep erythrocytes is significantly impaired in BRSV-infected cultures, but no differences are noted in macrophage viability, ability to adhere to glass, killing ability, latex bead phagocytosis, or lysosomal enzyme content.[33]

Macrophage/neutrophil interaction, as well as neutrophil function, may be impaired in calves exposed to an aerosol of BHV-1 virus initially and then to an aerosol of *P. haemolytica* 5 days later.[34] Analysis of sequential lavage fluids suggests that neutrophil infiltration into the lung is delayed in response to the presence of the bacteria. In vitro studies of these cells show neutrophils from infected animals display little random migration and do not respond to a chemotactic stimulus.[34] Macrophages are not able to produce neutrophil chemotactic factors.[34] Another BHV-1 aerosol challenge study notes significant depression of neutrophil chemotactic response but no significant effects on antibacterial activity.[35] A modified-live vaccine strain of BVDV administered intranasally or intramuscularly to cattle decreases the number of circulating neutrophils and suppresses iodination and neutrophil-mediated antibody-dependent cellular cytotoxicity.[36] Aerosol exposure to PI$_3$ significantly reduces chemiluminescence and iodination ability of neutrophils in calves; however, random migration, *Staphylococcus aureus* ingestion, cytochrome-*c* reduction, and antibody-dependent cellular cytotoxicity are not significantly affected by aerosol exposure to PI$_3$.[37]

A study examining interaction of BHV-1 and lymphocyte function demonstrates significant depression in lymphocyte blastogenic response to mitogens (a measure of the ability of lymphocytes to proliferate), as well as to *P. haemolytica* and *P. multocida*.[37] In vitro infection of lymphocytes with live BHV-1 inhibits blastogenic response of bovine blood mononuclear cells to a mitogen (phytohemagglutinin), whereas no effects are seen following infection with ultraviolet-irradiated BHV-1.[38] Intravenous inoculation of BHV-1 decreases the number of circulating lymphocytes by more than 50%.[39]

A variety of lymphocyte-suppressive phenomena are associated with BVDV. Administration of a modified-live vaccine strain of BVDV decreases the number of circulating lymphocytes and their response to mitogens.[36] In cattle persistently infected with BVDV, proliferative response of both resting and mitogen-stimulated blood mononuclear cells is suppressed.[40-42] Lymphocytes from calves experimentally infected intratracheally with PI$_3$ show reduced response to stimulation with phytohemagglutinin in blastogenesis assays. The effects are most severe between days 2 to 7 and gradually abate over days 8 to 10.[43]

Epidemiologic evidence suggests that viral immunosuppression leads to secondary bacterial pneumonia, yet understanding of specific immunosuppressive viral effects that cause this is incomplete. There is no information for many viruses isolated from bovine lungs, such as bovine adenovirus, bovine enterovirus, bovine parvovirus, coronavirus, calicivirus, bovine reovirus, bovine rhinovirus, malignant catarrhal fever virus, and bovine herpesvirus 4. In many cases, relevance of current in vitro tests to in vivo function is speculative. Tests are insufficient to evaluate many aspects of the host immune system, such as cytotoxic T lymphocytes.

The importance of *Chlamydia* spp., another obligate intracellular pathogen in bovine respiratory disease, is well characterized. The organism appears to inhibit alveolar macrophage killing at least well enough to facilitate its own survival.[44] Clinical disease resulting from experimental infection with *P. haemolytica* is more severe when *Chlamydia* is added to the challenge, suggesting respiratory defense suppression.[45]

Like viruses, mycoplasmas may contribute to the development of bovine respiratory disease. Evidence suggests that they compromise innate defenses, including the mucociliary escalator,[46] bovine alveolar macrophages,[47] and neutrophils.[48] Evidence also suggests that they have negative effects on the acquired immune system.[49,50]

P. haemolytica has at least two critical virulence factors.[51] It possesses a capsule that makes it difficult for leukocytes to phagocytize bacteria. Additionally, it produces an exotoxin (also called a cytotoxin or leukotoxin) that is lethal for ruminant leukocytes. Thus a major nonspecific host defense mechanism used against acute bacterial infection, the neutrophil, is severely compromised.

Virulence mechanisms and/or immunosuppressive effects of *H. somnus* are not as well characterized. Isolates from cattle with clinical disease are reportedly resistant to killing by complement in normal serum. This resistance is associated with the ability of other gram-negative bacteria to invade mammalian tissues[52] and may be associated with the composition of the bacterial surface. In an experiment involving challenge of a small number of calves, reintroduction of *H. somnus* lipopolysaccharide to a semipurified vaccine containing outer membrane antigens of *H. somnus* reduced the efficacy of the vaccine, suggesting that *H. somnus* lipopolysaccharide interfered with the immunologic response to other *H. somnus* antigens.[53]

Other Factors

Distress is an important factor in determining an animal's ability to fight infection and respond to vaccines. Distress arises from a variety of sources, including transport, nutritional changes, weaning, and han-

dling, among others. Speculation on the relationship between distressors and disease resistance has been ongoing for centuries. In the nineteenth century, Pasteur noted that placing a chicken's legs in cold water increased its susceptibility to anthrax.

A similar relationship is seen in cattle. Weaning reduces antibody production in response to vaccine.[54,55] Lymphocyte function is suppressed in transported calves.[56,57] Dehydration, resulting from cattle being without water (e.g., during transport), can decrease effectiveness of the tracheal cilia in clearing pathogens trapped in mucus from the respiratory tract. Castration is distressful and can decrease health and growth performance.[58–63] Increased cortisol levels are associated with many environmental and management factors, such as surgical castration[64,65] and dehorning.[66] Increased cortisol levels are associated with decreases in a variety of indicators of immune status.[57,67–70] Elevated cortisol levels resulting from physiologic or psychologic distressors negatively affect several neutrophil functions and depress lymphocyte proliferation.[71]

We should minimize distressors as much as possible to prevent compromise of host defense systems. The concept of additive distressors is especially relevant when discussing the immunologic sequelae of distress. Usually, it is not a single distressor that debilitates the immune system. More often, cumulative effects of a series of mild to moderate distressors experienced over a period of hours to days depress immune function below a threshold such that immune response is no longer effective. Not only does each animal have a unique immunologic history, but each animal varies in its response to distressors, resulting in the wide spectrum of morbidity and response to vaccination frequently seen in cattle.

Once the importance of additive distressors as well as that of the interactions between distress and immune function is appreciated, it becomes apparent that a positive intervention for health managers involves the identification and minimization of preventable distressors. Many distressors that cattle encounter result from the marketing and management systems inherent in the cattle industry in the United States. Often we can have little impact on such distressors. If we objectively examine our management strategies, however, we will see that we tolerate many controllable distressors in the interest of economics or convenience.

Genetic predisposition to disease occurs in other species and has been speculated to occur in cattle. One example is the recently described bovine leukocyte adhesion deficiency.[72] In this heritable condition, affected calves lack a protein on the neutrophil surface required for adherence to the wall of blood vessels—a step required before migration into tissues can occur. Affected cattle have very high numbers of neutrophils in circulation but a paucity in tissues. Such cattle succumb to any of a variety of common neonatal diseases and respond poorly to antibiotics, emphasizing the importance of an innate immune system for optimal antibiotic efficacy. In another example, cattle with certain interferon genotypes display more severe clinical signs following experimental exposure to BHV-1 than do calves with other interferon genotypes; this suggests that genetics partially determines the degree of clinical signs displayed.[73]

Passive transfer of maternal antibodies present in colostrum is an important event in preventing respiratory and other diseases early in a calf's life.[74] However, the impact on health and growth performance continues past weaning. One study indicates that calves with inadequate passive transfer as determined by 24 hour plasma protein levels are at greater risk of respiratory morbidity (odds ratio [OR] = 3.1) in the feedlot than are calves with adequate passive transfer.[75]

Age is another important host factor. The bovine immune system begins to develop during gestation.[76] Even though the bovine fetus is capable of recognizing and responding to antigens before birth, the immune system does not reach peak function until around puberty. During old age, immunocompetence wanes, although this is rarely of practical significance in feedlots.

A calf's previous nutritional status and parasite burden can affect its overall physiology and immune responsiveness. Parasites produce immunosuppressive substances as they progress through larval molts.[77] Nutritional deficiencies in energy and protein likely compromise overall physiology and immune function. Trace minerals and vitamins play an important role in maintaining optimal immune function, although this is incompletely understood and the practical implications are even move obscure.

PREVENTION

Sound husbandry and good management are key to maintaining immunocompetence. We can fall into the trap of relying on products as the solution for all problems. While these products may be valuable aids, they cannot replace sound animal care practices. This section discusses management strategies to prevent or reduce disease by preventing exposure of the calf to the pathogen, preventing infection of the calf by the pathogen, and by helping the calf fight infection by bolstering the acquired immune system.

Preventing Exposure

An obvious and important way to help the immune system is to prevent exposure. Many management strategies can help accomplish this. Examples are closed herd or screened replacements, sanitation, and vaccine herd effect.

With a closed herd, the opportunity for exposure to pathogens is reduced. Alternatively, new animals can be isolated and screened for disease prior to introduction to the herd. Unfortunately, neither of these approaches is practical in feedlots, making other means of reducing exposure, such as sanitation, even more important.

Sanitation is an often underemphasized

management tool. Pathogens are everywhere in the environment; although they can never be completely eliminated, their numbers can be reduced. The number of pathogens an animal encounters is a critical determinant of whether or not infection and disease will result. Space and sunlight can be useful tools to reduce pathogen numbers. Reducing animal density can decrease transmission events by reducing animal contacts; sunlight kills many pathogens. Other strategies—such as keeping receiving pens, hospital areas, and the like as clean as feasible—require dedication and attention to detail.

Another way to prevent exposure of susceptible animals to disease agents is through herd immunity. Herd immunity is based on the fact that transmission of communicable disease requires contact between infectious individuals (i.e., those that are shedding virus) and susceptible ones. Raising resistance in a herd by natural exposure or vaccination reduces the number of susceptible animals and the number of infected animals during an outbreak, thereby reducing the number of contacts between susceptible and infectious animals. This indirectly protects all the susceptible animals, especially in outbreaks of highly contagious disease.

Our goal in herd immunization is to raise the level of immunity in a sufficient number of animals to prevent epidemics and the catastrophic monetary losses associated with them. In this approach, individual animals may still become ill, especially if other factors that reduce disease resistance are present. In a population of immune animals, disease transmission decreases as resistance to disease increases. This reduces, but does not eliminate, occurrence of diseases with high morbidity or mortality. Paradoxically, individual animals can still become ill even when a vaccine successfully stimulates an effective level of herd immunity.

Preventing Infection

Although exposure may occur, infection and disease do not necessarily follow. The animal encounters pathogens every day

of its life, but only rarely does it become ill. The agent must infect the animal to cause disease. As previously discussed, the animal has several defenses designed to prevent this event.

An important concept to remember is that many of the prevention strategies mentioned above are influenced only by husbandry, not by vaccines. Vaccines influence herd effect, antibodies in mucus, and antibodies and lymphocytes mobilized to action *after* viral and/or bacterial invasion occurs.

Immunization

Vaccine-induced immunity is one of several management tools available to help achieve optimum livestock productivity through disease prevention, control, and eradication. Disease surveillance is critical to each herd program to determine need and to evaluate the effectiveness of each immunization procedure. This surveillance requires accurate monitoring of clinically affected animals and postmortem examination of all dead calves.

Two key components required for successful immunization are an efficacious vaccine and an immunocompetent animal (i.e., an animal with a functioning immune system; also referred to as an immunologically competent animal). Along with challenge dose considerations, these form the basis for vaccination success. Vaccine failures arise from inattention to details in these critical areas (as discussed later in the section on optimizing immunizations).

Acquired immunity is mediated by lymphocytes. Lymphocytes, along with some accessory cells, are responsible for recognizing foreign substances, responding to them, producing soluble factors such as interleukin and interferon, killing infected and foreign cells, and producing antibodies. In contrast to innate defenses, acquired defenses are antigen specific and antigen driven and are mediated by antibodies, cytotoxic T lymphocytes, and cytokines produced during an immune response.

The acquired immune response consists of three phases: cognition, activation, and effector.[78] Depending on the immuno-logic experience of the animal, these phases take a varying number of days to occur, with maximum response seen 2 to 4 weeks after antigen exposure.

The acquired immune response is initiated by recognition of a foreign substance (also called an antigen). This can be a virus, bacteria, toxin, or any other nonself substance. During the cognition phase, antigen-presenting cells process and present the antigen to lymphocytes for recognition.

The activation phase is the sequence of immune events that occur as a result of the cognition phase. Lymphocytes undergo two major changes in response to antigens: (1) they proliferate, leading to expansion of the clones of antigen-specific lymphocytes and amplification of the immune response, and (2) they differentiate to cells that eliminate foreign antigens.

During the effector phase, antigen-activated lymphocytes eliminate the antigen through functions such as antibody production by B lymphocytes and destruction of infected cells by cytotoxic T lymphocytes.

Different subtypes of lymphocytes have specific functions in the overall immune response. Some, called helper cells, are responsible for producing and releasing factors that enhance the immune response. Others, called suppressor cells, are able to decrease the immune response. The balance between the number and/or the net effects of these two cell types (the helper/suppressor ratio) is important in determining the animal's ability to respond to a vaccine. Certain lymphocytes are able to recognize and destroy cells infected by viruses or bacteria. These killer or cytotoxic cells are important in an animal's ability to fight intracellular infections. Helper, suppressor, and cytotoxic cells are all part of the cell-mediated immune system and are included in the general classification of T lymphocytes, as they come from the thymus.

The term "cell-mediated immunity" can have several meanings, especially with regard to modified-live and killed vaccines. Inconsistent usage of this term has resulted in confusion. In its most general sense, cell-mediated immunity can include any immune phenomenon mediated by a cell. More specifically, it can be used to refer to only those effects mediated by cytotoxic T lymphocytes. Most commonly, it is used to describe any effect mediated by T lymphocytes, including T helper, T suppressor, and T cytotoxic cells. During the activation stage of the immune response, a T helper cell response is a necessary part of antibody production by B lymphocytes.

Indirect measures of immune function that assess T helper cell function, such as lymphoproliferation, are likely to show a positive response even if the effector component of cell-mediated immunity, cytotoxic T lymphocytes, is not stimulated. For example, following administration of modified-live BHV-1 vaccine to a naive animal, virus replication occurs and the immune system responds to this "infection" as outlined above. T helper cells are activated, cytokines are produced, antibody titer rises, and cytotoxic T lymphocytes "see" virus-infected cells and are primed. In response to killed vaccine, all of this occurs as well, except that the immune system is not exposed to virally infected cells. Practical implications of these differences vary among pathogens and are difficult to assess. The differences may partially account for variations noted in immune responses to modified-live versus killed virus vaccines.

The cells responsible for producing antibodies are called B lymphocytes. When a foreign substance is presented to B lymphocytes, they recognize it (cognition phase) and undergo repeated divisions, eventually maturing into antigen-specific, antibody-producing lymphocytes (activation phase). The increased number of activated lymphocytes producing antibodies results in an increased antibody titer to the inducing antigen (effect phase). This increase in antibody titer is used to evaluate effectiveness of a vaccine; however, as briefly discussed, antibody response comprises only one part of a very complex process.

Optimizing Immunization

For a vaccine to work, the immune response that it elicits must occur prior to challenge. If a vaccine is used in any fashion other than prior to exposure, vaccine efficacy will be suboptimal or negligible.

Preexposure vaccination, while not a panacea, has proven beneficial. In a review of controlled studies of the effect of preconditioning on feedlot health performance, morbidity is reduced from 26.5% to 20.4% and mortality is reduced from 1.44% to 0.74%.[79] The same report reviews survey reports and cites a reduction of 20% to 30% in morbidity and 0 to 1.7% in mortality.

What we know about how the immune system functions, along with the data cited above, supports the concept that the preexposure immunization component of preconditioning reduces morbidity and mortality (given the qualifiers listed below). Preconditioning does not eliminate disease. Morbidity and mortality rates in preconditioned calves are rarely zero. Thus, without a valid control group, it can be difficult to know the true value of preconditioning. Similarly, if no disease occurs in a given group, it is not possible to show a benefit. A final consideration is cost effectiveness. Even if it is assumed that preexposure immunization usually results in statistically significant reductions in morbidity and mortality rates, this does not necessarily mean that such treatment is cost effective. Economic considerations (e.g., cost of vaccine, cost of additional handling, and the like) must be weighed.

As stated initially, vaccination only ensures that the animal has been exposed to the antigens contained in that vaccine, not that a protective immune response has ensued. If either of the two previously discussed key components that are required for a successful immunization—an efficacious vaccine and an immunocompetent animal—is missing, the result will be apparent failure of the vaccine.

Achieving a protective immune response to every pathogen in every animal in a population is probably impossible for several reasons. Even if it could be achieved, it would likely be cost prohibitive. Based on the pathogenesis of the specific organism, some vaccines need to achieve immunity in each individual in a population for the products to be efficacious. An example is an infectious, but noncommunicable, disease such as tetanus. In the case of other pathogens, especially those that are highly contagious, reducing the number of susceptible animals below a critical threshold may be sufficient for the vaccine to prevent a disease outbreak (the concept of herd immunity).

A vaccine may seem ineffective if it does not contain antigens that induce protective immunity to the disease-causing agent currently challenging the calf. No vaccines are available for some respiratory pathogens that can influence calf health, such as *Chlamydia* spp.[46] Antigenic differences among strains and species of pathogens or changes in antigens the organism displays may compromise vaccine efficacy, as illustrated by the genetic and antigenic instability of BVDV.[80] This instability was thought to contribute to the failure of repeated annual doses of inactivated virus vaccine to protect animals from infection.[81] For many infectious agents of cattle, however, immunologically important antigens are relatively stable.

A more likely cause of vaccine ineffectiveness is improper handling, as described in the discussion of BHV-1. Vaccines must be stored and administered according to recommendations; otherwise, there is a risk that their efficacy will be reduced. Special care must be taken with a live vaccine, either viral or bacterial, to prevent inactivating the vaccine by exposing it to extremes in temperature, ultraviolet radiation, disinfectants, and the like.

Once it is ensured that the vaccine and the equipment have been cared for properly, the vaccine must be carefully administered. Training sessions should be conducted to ensure that personnel are knowledgeable about the proper locations and techniques for vaccine administration.[82] Intramuscular injections should not be made behind the calf's front leg. The subcutaneous route should be used whenever label instructions allow. As a general rule, the smallest needle through which the product is easily delivered should be used. For thin, watery products, an 18 gauge needle works well. Needle length should be adjusted for calf size and injection route. Give intramuscular injections with a 1½ inch needle; however, a 1 inch needle should be used for small calves. Make subcutaneous injections with a ½ or ⅝ inch needle. Change needles after 10 injections or whenever they become dull, barbed, or bent. Use a clean needle when refilling syringes to avoid contaminating the vaccine bottle. Good handling facilities help minimize injection site reactions by ensuring that cattle are adequately restrained to prevent movement if a struggle ensues during an injection.

Sanitation is an important component of any vaccination plan and helps minimize injection site reactions and abscesses. Contamination of a multidose container can result in vaccine inactivation and injection site problems. Disinfectants inactivate modified-live vaccines, so care must be taken to properly clean and rinse all equipment that comes in contact with vaccine.

Timing of vaccine administration can also influence the perception of effectiveness. If a disease is in the incubation phase or if exposure to a disease-causing agent occurs soon after vaccination, an animal may become ill and the vaccine will appear ineffective. It takes several days for the immune system to mount a protective response following vaccination, especially if a calf is immunologically naive.

Experimentally, if enough disease-causing organisms are given, disease is induced even in immune animals. When cattle are assembled in close quarters, the amount of disease agent to which they are exposed may be quite large, resulting in disease even in immune animals. As discussed previously, there are several management steps to counter this.

Individual animal responsiveness can affect success or failure of vaccination. Not all animals are able to respond to vaccines for a variety of reasons already mentioned, including age, nutrition, genetics, stress, and previous vaccination/disease history.

Vaccines

Both live and killed vaccines are available. The advantages of one usually balance the disadvantages of the other. Attributes of modified-live vaccine include:

- Strong, long-lasting immune response achieved with fewer doses
- Less reliance on adjuvants
- Possible stimulation of interferon production by viral vaccines
- Stimulation of the effector component of cell-mediated immunity (cytotoxic T lymphocytes)
- The bacteria or virus contained in the vaccine resembling the pathogenic form of the organism more closely

Killed vaccines also have certain advantages:

- More stable in storage
- Unlikely to cause disease due to residual virulence or reversion of virulence

Numerous vaccine products provide a variety of combinations of live and/or killed antigens. These include BHV-1, BVDV, PI$_3$, BRSV, *Pasteurella* spp., and *H. somnus*. Reviews of these vaccines and their usage are available.[52,83]

BHV-1 vaccines are offered in modified-live virus form for intramuscular, subcutaneous, or intranasal use. Killed and chemically altered viral products are available for intramuscular use. Intramuscular modified-live virus vaccines quickly induce long-lasting immunity following proper administration of a single dose.[84,85] Intranasal modified-live virus vaccines induce immunity at the mucosal surface through stimulation of acquired mucosal immunity and production of interferon.[86,87] They may be used safely in calves suckling pregnant cows and induce immunity in the face of residual maternal antibody titers. However, they are more difficult to administer. Killed virus vaccines require administration of two doses at a 14 to 28 day interval to induce immunity, have a higher cost, and provide a shorter duration of immunity, making them less practical to use in a typical feedlot setting.

BVDV vaccines are available in modified-live and killed virus forms and constitute one of the most controversial vaccines in U.S. feedlots. Lack of large scale efficacy trials, widespread BVDV infection in the U.S. cattle population, presence of persistently infected cattle that subsequently develop mucosal disease, and the emerging role of heterologous and novel strains of the virus all contribute to the controversy.[83,88] There is no clear consensus concerning usage. Measurements of certain immune parameters suggest that immunosuppression following use of modified-live virus may be of concern[37]; however, the lack of complications following use in large numbers of cattle suggests that these may be of no practical concern.[89] Modified-live BVDV vaccines may be of greater concern in highly stressed cattle, but well-controlled studies evaluating this are not available. As with the BHV-1 products, dosage and timing requirements of killed BVDV vaccines are a severe limitation in most feedlot settings.

BRSV vaccines are available in modified-live and inactivated virus forms. Since recovery from natural infection with respiratory syncytial virus does not engender protective immunity in most species, it is unlikely that vaccination will prevent subsequent infection.[90] However, it may still be possible for vaccination to attenuate clinical signs of subsequent infections and decrease the time to recovery. One experimental challenge of a small number of calves shows that passive antibodies reduce the pathology associated with BRSV.[91] In a random, double-blind study comparing morbidity rates in cattle receiving two doses of a vaccine containing BRSV to those receiving two doses of a similar vaccine without

BRSV, cattle receiving vaccine that did not contain BRSV were 1.4 times more likely to be ill (Yates corrected chi-square p-value = 0.00002).[92] Other reports of efficacy have used either historical controls[93] or have relied on numerical differences that were not statistically significant.[94] There are reports of improvement in gain and feed efficiency.[95] These mixed reports of efficacy make the use of BRSV vaccines controversial but suggest that they may be useful in naive, weaned calves.

Studies show PI$_3$ virus compromises innate defenses of the respiratory tract.[96,97] Because many older cattle arriving at feedlots are likely immune, the value of vaccinating yearling cattle is questionable. Vaccination may be beneficial in preweaning or arrival programs involving less immunologically experienced calves. As a practical matter, it is difficult to select a multivirus bovine respiratory vaccine that does not include PI$_3$.

Research indicates that the newer *Pasteurella* vaccines, which induce antibodies against both capsular and cytotoxin antigens, reduce respiratory morbidity when used rationally.[79,98,99] Because of dosage and timing requirements for optimal immunity (optimal immunity occurs 7 to 10 days following a booster dose given 14 to 21 days after the primary dose), their value is compromised when used only in a feedlot arrival program.

Ability of *H. somnus* vaccine to reduce bovine respiratory disease in U.S. feedlots may be limited by the low incidence and sporadic nature of infection with this pathogen.[100] While studies demonstrate vaccine efficacy, most have involved septicemic challenge.[101] Some have shown efficacy in experimental respiratory challenge.[102,103] To date, however, efficacy has not been unequivocally demonstrated in well-controlled trials in a U.S. field setting.[83] These vaccines suffer from the same dose and timing requirements of *Pasteurella* vaccines.

CARCASS QUALITY

Raising cattle is, in effect, producing food, so maintaining product quality is a high priority. Consequently, proper use and administration of animal health products to food animals are vitally important. Carcass damage frequently occurs when biologic compounds are administered without close attention to proper technique. Such damage may not be apparent to the livestock producer or even the packer. However, recent surveys suggest that damaged tissue found during fabrication represents a loss of millions of dollars to the cattle industry. Some reports estimate injection damage to the top sirloin area alone costs $1.74 per head processed, or $35.7 million annually.[105] In the long run, producers bear the brunt of these costs as reflected in the bids for their livestock. Injection techniques should be considered from the perspective of the animal as well. Industry professionals must remind producers to read and follow label directions, be clean, and use the technique recommendations listed above. Veterinarians need to serve as positive role models when administering any biologic compound; this is extremely important as it is easy to become complacent when performing everyday procedures. If veterinarians deliver a high standard of practice, it is easier to demand high standards from producers.

SUMMARY

Specific vaccine recommendations should be made by the veterinarian familiar with the management of the operation, including type of cattle handled and disease problems typically experienced. There are few cookbook solutions. Fine-tuning each program by including or excluding certain vaccines requires us to identify the specific disease entities present in an operation. This requires good records, complete postmortem examinations, and a good diagnostic support system. Effective management to optimize the animals' immunocompetence and timing of vaccine administration is as important as selecting the correct vaccine product.

From an immunologic standpoint, optimum control of pneumonia in feedlot cattle begins with effective management of passive transfer in newborn calves, followed by rational and proper vaccine use in preconditioning programs. Control continues through maintenance of innate pulmonic defenses by minimizing time in market channels, choosing to manage cattle in a manner that eliminates or minimizes as many physical and behavioral distressors as possible, and, to the extent possible, minimizing unnecessary exposure to pathogens.

REFERENCES

1. Corstvet RE, Panciera RJ, Rinker HB, et al: Survey of tracheas of feedlot cattle for *Hemophilus somnus* and other selected bacteria. *JAVMA* 163:870, 1973.
2. Yates WDG: A review of infectious bovine rhinotracheitis, shipping fever pneumonia and viral-bacterial synergism in respiratory disease of cattle. *Can J Comp Med* 46:225, 1982.
3. Butler JE: Bovine immunoglobulins: An augmented review. *Vet Immunol Immunopathol* 4:43, 1982.
4. Jakab GJ: Viral-bacterial interactions in respiratory tract infections: A review of the mechanisms of virus-induced suppression of pulmonary antibacterial defenses, in Loan RW (ed) : *Bovine Respiratory Disease, A Symposium*. College Station, TX, Texas A&M University Press, 1984, p 223.
5. Babiuk LA, Acres SD: Models for bovine respiratory disease, in Loan RW (ed): *Bovine Respiratory Disease, A Symposium*. College Station, TX, Texas A&M University Press, 1984, p 287.
6. Mims CA: Microbial strategies, in *Pathogenesis of Infectious Disease*. New York, Academic Press, 1982, p 135.
7. Jericho KWF, Langford EV: Pneumonia in calves produced with aerosols of bovine herpes virus I and *Pasteurella haemolytica. Can J Comp Med* 42:269, 1978.
8. Jericho KWF: Histological changes in the respiratory tract of calves exposed to aerosols of bovine herpesvirus I and *Pasteurella hemolytica. J Comp Pathol* 93:73, 1983.
9. Yates WDG, Jericho KWF, Doige CE: Effect of viral dose on experimental pneumonia caused by aerosol exposure of calves to bovine herpesvirus 1 and *Pasteurella haemolytica. Can J Comp Med* 47:57, 1983.
10. Yates WDG, Babiuk LA, Jericho KWF: Pneumonia in calves: Duration of the interaction between bovine herpesvirus I and *Pasteurella haemolytica. Can J Comp Med* 47:257, 1983.
11. Yates WDG, Jericho KWF, Doige CE: Effect

of bacterial dose on pneumonia induced by aerosol exposure of calves to bovine herpesvirus-l and *Pasteurella haemolytica. Am J Vet Res* 44:238, 1983.

12. Frank GH, Briggs RE, Gillette KG: Colonization of the nasal passages of calves with *Pasteurella hemolytica* serotype 1 and regeneration of colonization after experimentally induced viral infection of the respiratory tract. *Am J Vet Res* 47:1704, 1986.

13. Hamoud M, Imrey PB, Woods GT, et al: An epidemiologic study of acute respiratory disease in beef calves after weaning. *Bovine Pract* 2:7, 1981.

14. Corstvet RE, Panciera RJ: Effect of infectious bovine rhinotracheitis virus and bovine virus diarrhea virus on *Pasteurella haemolytica* infection in the bovine lung. *Proc Am Assoc Vet Lab Diag* 25:363, 1982.

15. Baldwin DE, Marshall RG, Wessman GE: Experimental infection of calves with myxovirus parainfluenza-3 and *Pasteurella haemolytica. Am J Vet Res* 28:1773, 1967.

16. Trapp AL, Hamdy AH, Gale C, et al: Lesions in calves exposed to agents associated with the shipping fever complex. *Am J Vet Res* 27:1235, 1966.

17. Jericho KWF, Darcel CQ, Langford EV: Respiratory disease in calves produced with aerosols of parainfluenza-3 virus and *Pasteurella haemolytica. Can J Comp Med* 46:293, 1982.

18. Heddleston KL, Reisinger RC, Watko LP: Studies on the transmission and etiology of bovine shipping fever. *Am J Vet Res* 23:548, 1962.

19. Hetrick FM, Chang SC, Byrne RJ, et al: The combined effect of *Pasteurella multocida* and myxovirus parainfluenza-3 upon calves. *Am J Vet Res* 24:939, 1963.

20. Bohlender RE, McCune MW, Frey ML: Bovine respiratory syncytial virus infection. *Mod Vet Pract* 3:613, 1982.

21. Lehmkuhl LD, Gough PM: Investigation of causative agents of bovine respiratory tract disease in a beef cow-calf herd with an early weaning program. *Am J Vet Res* 38:1717, 1977.

22. Rossi CR, Kiesel GK: Susceptibility of bovine macrophage and tracheal-ring cultures to bovine viruses. *Am J Vet Res* 38:1705, 1977.

23. Allen EM, Msolla PM: Scanning electron microscopy of the tracheal epithelium of calves inoculated with bovine herpesvirus I. *Res Vet Sci* 29:325, 1980.

24. Rossi CR, Kiesel GK: Susceptibility of bovine macrophage and tracheal-ring cultures to bovine viruses. *Am J Vet Res* 38:1705, 1977.

25. Gilka F, Thomson RG, Savan M: The effect of edema, hydrocortisone acetate, concurrent viral infection and immunization on the clearance of *Pasteurella hemolytica* from the bovine lung. *Can J Comp Med* 38:251, 1976.

26. Lopex A, Thomson RG, Savan M: The pulmonary clearance of *Pasteurella hemolytica* in calves infected with bovine parainfluenza-3 virus. *Can J Comp Med* 40:385, 1976.

27. Al-Izzi SA, Maxie MG, Savan M: The pulmonary clearance of *Pasteurella haemolytica* in calves given *Corynebacterium parvum* and infected with parainfluenza-3 virus. *Can J Comp Med* 46:85, 1982.

28. Castleman WL, Chandler SK, Slauson DO: Experimental bovine respiratory syncytial virus infection in conventional calves: Ultrastructural respiratory lesions. *Am J Vet Res* 46:554, 1985.

29. Toth TN, Hesse RA: Replication of five bovine respiratory viruses in cultured bovine alveolar macrophages. *Arch Virol* 75:219, 1983.

30. Forman AJ, Babiuk LA, Misra V, et al: Susceptibility of bovine macrophages to infectious bovine rhinotracheitis virus infection. *Infect Immun* 35:1048, 1982.

31. Forman AJ, Babiuk LA: Effect of infectious bovine rhinotracheitis virus infection on bovine alveolar macrophage function. *Infect Immun* 35:1041, 1982.

32. Hesse RA, Toth TE: Effects of bovine parainfluenza-3 virus on phagocytosis and phagosome-lysosome fusion of cultured bovine alveolar macrophages. *Am J Vet Res* 44:1901, 1983.

33. Trigo E, Liggitt HD, Evermann JF, et al: Effect of *in vitro* inoculation of bovine respiratory syncytial virus on bovine pulmonary alveolar macrophage function. *Am J Vet Res* 46:1098, 1985.

34. McGuire RL, Babiuk LA: Evidence for defective neutrophil function in lungs of calves exposed to infectious bovine rhinotracheitis virus. *Vet Immunol Immunopathol* 5:259, 1984.

35. Filion, LG, McGuire RL, Babiuk LA: Nonspecific suppressive effect of bovine herpesvirus type I on bovine leukocyte function. *Infect Immun* 42:106, 1983.

36. Roth JA, Kaeberle ML: Suppression of neutrophil and lymphocyte function induced by a vaccinal strain of bovine viral diarrhea virus with and without the administration of ACTH. *Am J Vet Res* 44:2366, 1983.

37. Briggs RE, Kehrli M, Frank GH: Effects of infection with parainfluenza-3 virus and infectious bovine rhinotracheitis virus on neutrophil functions in calves. *Am J Vet Res* 49:682, 1988.

38. Pollard A, Magnuson NS, Yilma T, et al: Suppression of the bovine mitogenic response by

infectious bovine rhinotracheitis (IBR) virus. *Fed Proc* 44:529, 1985 (abstract).

39. Cummins JM, Rosenquist BD: Leukocyte changes and interferon production in calves injected with hydrocortisone and infected with infectious bovine rhinotracheitis virus. *Am J Vet Res* 40:238, 1979.

40. Roth JA, Kaeberle ML, Griffith RW: Effects of bovine viral diarrhea virus infection on bovine polymorphonuclear leukocyte function. *Am J Vet Res* 42:244, 1981.

41. Bolin SR, Roth JA, Uhlenhopp EK, et al: Immunologic and virologic findings in a bull chronically infected with noncytopathic bovine viral diarrhea virus. *JAVMA* 190:1015, 1987.

42. Johnson DW, Muscoplat CC: Immunologic abnormalities in calves with chronic bovine viral diarrhea. *Am J Vet Res* 34:1139, 1973.

43. Pospisil Z, Machatkova M, Mensik J, et al: Decline in the phytohemagglutinin responsiveness of lymphocytes from calves infected experimentally with bovine viral diarrhoea-mucosal disease virus and parainfluenza 3 virus. *ACTA Vet BRNO* 44:369, 1975.

44. Eissenberg LG, Wyrick P: Inhibition of phagolysosome fusion is localized to *Chlamydia psittaci*-laden vacuoles. *Infect Immun* 32:889, 1981.

45. Palotay JL, Christensen NR: Bovine respiratory infection I. Psittacosis-lymphogranuloma venereum group of viruses as etiological agents. *JAVMA* 134:222, 1959.

46. Jarstrand C, Camner P, Philipson K: *Mycoplasma pneumoniae* tracheobronchial clearance. *Am Rev Resp Dis* 110:41, 1975.

47. Almeida RA, Wannemuehler MJ, Rosenbusch RF: Interaction of *Mycoplasma dispar* with bovine alveolar macrophages. *Infect Immun* 60:2914, 1992.

48. Thomas CB, Van Ess P, Wolfgram LJ, et al: Adherence to bovine neutrophils and suppression of neutrophil chemiluminescence by *Mycoplasma bovis*. *Vet Immunol Immunopathol* 27:365, 1991.

49. Bennett RH, Jasper DE: Immunosuppression of humoral and cell-mediated responses in calves associated with inoculation of *Mycoplasma bovis*. *Am J Vet Res* 38:1731, 1977.

50. Finch JM, Howard CL: Inhibitory effect of *M. dispar* and *M. bovis* on bovine immune responses *in vitro,* in Stanek G, Cassell G, Tully JG, et al (eds): *Recent Advances in Mycoplasmology.* New York, Gustav Fischer Verlag, 1990, p 563.

51. Mosier DA, Confer AW, Panciera RJ: The evolution of vaccines for bovine pneumonic pasteurellosis. *Res Vet Sci* 47:1, 1989.

52. Corbeil LB, Widders PR, Gogolewski R, Arthur J, et al: *Haemophilus somnus:* Bovine reproductive and respiratory disease. *Can Vet J* 27:90, 1986.

53. Silva SVPS, Little PB: The protective effect of vaccination against experimental pneumonia in cattle with *Haemophilus somnus* outer membrane antigens and interference by lipopolysaccharide. *Can J Vet Res* 54:326, 1990.

54. Gwazdauskas FC, Gross WB, Bibb TL, et al: Antibody titers and plasma glucocorticoid concentrations near weaning in steer and heifer calves. *Can Vet J* 19:150, 1978.

55. Pollock JM, Rowan TG, Dixon JB, et al: Effects of weaning on antibody responses in young calves. *Vet Immunol Immunopathol* 33:25, 1992.

56. Filion LG, Willson PJ, Bielefeldt-Ohmann H, et al: The possible role of stress in the induction of pneumonic pasteurellosis. *Can J Comp Med* 48:268, 1984.

57. Blecha F, Boyles SL, Riles JG: Shipping suppresses lymphocytes blastogenic responses in Angus and Brahman x Angus feeder calves. *J Anim Sci* 59:576, 1984.

58. Lofgreen GP, Addis DG, Dunbar JR, et al: Time of processing calves subjected to marketing and shipping stress. *J Anim Sci* 47:132, 1978.

59. Zinn RA, Dunbar JR, Norman BB: Relative effects of dehorning and castration on early health and performance of feedlot calves. California Feeder's Day, 1985, p 97.

60. Worrell MA, Clanton DC, Calkins CR: Effect of weight at castration on steer performance in the feedlot. *J Anim Sci* 64:34, 1987.

61. Brazle FK: Effect of long-acting penicillin and levamisole on gain and health of stocker calves purchased as steers or bulls. *Agri-Practice* 13:8, 1992.

62. Zweiacher ER, Durham RM, Boren BD, et al: Effects of method and time of castration of feeder calves. *J Anim Sci* 49:5, 1979.

63. Faulkner DB, Eurell T, Tranquilli WJ, et al: Performance and health of weanling bulls after butorphanol and xylazine administration at castration. *J Anim Sci* 70:2970, 1992.

64. Thomas LR, Cohen RDH, Janzen ED, et al: Effect of method of castration on physiological stress in cattle. *J Anim Sci* 61(Suppl 1):394, 1985.

65. Fell LR, Shutt DA: Use of salivary cortisol as an indicator of stress due to management practices in sheep and calves. *Proc Aust Soc Anim Prod* 16:203, 1986.

66. Laden SA, Wohlt JE, Zajac PK, et al: Effects of stress from electrical dehorning on feed intake, growth, and blood constituents of Holstein heifer calves. *J Dairy Sci* 68:3062, 1985.

67. Roth JA: Immunosuppression and immunomodulation in bovine respiratory disease, in Loan RW (ed): *Bovine Respiratory Dis-*

ease, A Symposium. College Station, TX, Texas A&M University Press, 1984, p 143.

68. Kelley KW: Immunological consequences of changing environmental stimuli. *Anim Stress* 1985, p 193.

69. Gwazdauskas FC, Gross WB, Bibb TL, et al: Antibody titers and plasma glucocorticoid concentrations near weaning in steer and heifer calves. *Can Vet J* 19:150, 1978.

70. Murata H, Takahashi H, Matsumoto H: The effect of road transportation on peripheral blood lymphocyte subpopulations, lymphocyte blastogenesis and neutrophil function in calves. *Br Vet J* 143:166, 1987.

71. Roth JA: Susceptibility to bovine respiratory disease, in *Proceedings of a Bovine Respiratory Disease Seminar.* Lawrenceville, NJ, Veterinary Learning Systems, 1987, p 4.

72. Gilbert RO, Rebhun WC, Kim CA: Clinical manifestations of leukocyte adhesion deficiency in cattle: 14 cases (1977–1991). *JAVMA* 202:445, 1993.

73. Ryan AM, Hutcheson DP, Womack JE: Type-I interferon genotypes and severity of clinical disease in cattle inoculated with bovine herpesvirus 1. *Am J Vet Res* 54:73, 1993.

74. Perino LJ, Sutherland RL, Woollen NE: Serum γ-glutamyltransferase activity and protein concentration at birth and after suckling in calves with adequate and inadequate passive transfer of immunoglobulin. *Am J Vet Res* 54:73, 1993.

75. Wittum TE, Perino LJ: Passive immune status at 24 hours postpartum and long-term health and performance of calves. *Am J Vet Res,* accepted for publication, 1995.

76. Schultz RD, Dunne HW, Heist CE: Ontogeny of the bovine immune response. *J Dairy Sci* 54:1321, 1974.

77. Gasbarre LC, Romanowski RD, Douvres FW: Suppression of antigen- and mitogen-induced proliferation of bovine lymphocytes by excretory-secretory products of *Oesophagostumum radiatum. Infect Immun* 48:540, 1985.

78. Abbas AK, Lichtman AH, Pober JS: General properties of immune responses, in *Cellular and Molecular Immunology.* Philadelphia, WB Saunders, 1991, p 4.

79. Cole NA: Preconditioning calves for the feedlot. *Vet Clin North Am Food Anim Pract* 1:401, 1985.

80. Corapi WV, Donis RO, Dubovi EJ: Characterization of a panel of monoclonal antibodies and their use in the study of the antigenic diversity of bovine viral diarrhea virus. *Am J Vet Res* 51:1388, 1990.

81. Kelling CL, Stine LC, Rump KK, et al: Investigation of bovine viral diarrhea virus infections in a range beef cattle herd. *JAVMA* 197:589, 1990.

82. Hudson DB, Perino LJ: Proper injection procedures for cattle. University of Nebraska NebGuide G92-1082-A.

83. Hjerpe CA: Bovine vaccines and herd vaccination programs. *Vet Clin North Am Food Anim Pract* 6:171, 1990.

84. Bordt DE, Thomas PC, Marshall RF: Early protection against infectious bovine rhinotracheitis with intramuscularly administered vaccine. *Proceedings of the 79th Annual Meeting of the US Animal Health Association* 79:50, 1975.

85. Sutton ML: Rapid onset of immunity in cattle after intramuscular injection of a modified live virus IBR vaccine. *Vet Med Small Anim Clin* 75:1447, 1980.

86. Cummins JM, Rosenquist BD: Leukocyte changes and interferon production in calves injected with hydrocortisone and infected with infectious bovine rhinotracheitis virus. *Am J Vet Res* 40:238, 1979.

87. Todd JD, Volenec FJ, Paton IM: Interferon on nasal secretions and sera of calves after intranasal administration of a virulent infectious bovine rhinotracheitis virus: Association of interferon in nasal secretions with early resistance to challenge with virulent virus. *Infect Immun* 5:699, 1972.

88. Radostits OM, Littlejohns IR: New concepts in the pathogenesis, diagnosis, and control of diseases caused by the bovine viral diarrhea virus. *Can Vet J* 29:513, 1988.

89. Edwards AJ: The effect of stressors like rumen overload and induced abortion on BRD in feedlot cattle. *Agri-Practice* 10:10, 1989.

90. Baker JC, Velicer LF: Bovine respiratory syncytial virus vaccination: Current status and future vaccine development. *Compend Contin Educ Pract Vet* 13:1323, 1991.

91. Bleknap EB, Baker JC, Patterson JS, Walker RD, et al: The role of passive immunity in bovine respiratory syncytial virus-infected calves. *J Infect Dis* 163:470, 1991.

92. Hansen DE, Syvrud R, Armstrong D: Effectiveness of a bovine respiratory syncytial virus vaccine in reducing the risk of respiratory disease. *Agri-Practice* 13: 19, 1992.

93. Syvrud R: Vaccination for bovine respiratory syncytial virus: Benefits for both cow/calf herd and feedlot cattle. *Proc AABP* 21:204, 1989.

94. Morter RL, Amstutz HE: Effectiveness of vaccination of feedlot cattle with bovine respiratory syncytial virus (BRSV). *Bovine Pract* 21:65, 1986.

95. Armstrong DA: Conclusion. *Proc Acad Vet Consultants,* p 62, Aug 27, 1987.

96. Reed SE, Boyd A: Organ cultures of respiratory epithelium infected with rhinovirus or parainfluenza virus studied in a scanning electron microscope. *Infect Immun* 6:68, 1972.

97. Lopez A, Thompson RG, Savan M: Pulmonary clearance of *P. hemolytica* in calves infected with bovine PI3 virus. *Can J Comp Med* 40:385, 1976.

98. Confer AW, Panciera RJ, Mosier DA: Bovine pneumonic pasteurellosis: Immunity to *Pasteurella haemolytica*. *JAVMA* 193:1308, 1988.

99. Bechtol DR, Ballinger RT, Sharp AJ: Field trial of a *Pasteurella haemolytica* toxoid administered at spring branding and in the feedlot. *Agri-Practice* 12:6, 1991.

100. Hjerpe CA: Clinical management of respiratory disease in feedlot cattle. *Vet Clin North Am Large Anim Pract* 5:119, 1983.

101. Stephens LR, Little PB, Wilkie BN, et al: Isolation of *Haemophilus somnus* antigens and their use as vaccines for prevention of bovine thromboembolic meningoencephalitis. *Am J Vet Res* 45:234, 1984.

102. Groom SC, Little PB: Effects of vaccination of calves against induced *Haemophilus somnus* pneumonia. *Am J Vet Res* 49:793, 1988.

103. Cairns R, Chu HJ, Chaves LJ, et al: Efficacy of an outer membrane complex *Haemophilus somnus* bacterin in preventing symptoms following *Haemophilus somnus* challenge. *Agri-Practice* 14:35, 1993.

104. National Cattlemen's Association National Beef Quality Audit, 1992.

Diagnostics for Bovine Respiratory Disease

Robert D. Glock, DVM, PhD, Professor
Veterinary Diagnostic Laboratories
Colorado State University
Fort Collins, Colorado

DIAGNOSTIC OBJECTIVES

A number of decisions must be made with regard to the effort dedicated to diagnosis of the various components and types of bovine respiratory disease (BRD). Economics often dictate the extent of effort and the type of procedures to be used. The ultimate objective must be health management through disease control. Mere development and proliferation of information may be interesting, but it is largely impractical if it cannot be applied to risk management. Ultimately, the reason we need to know the cause of disease is to help manage the disease more efficiently with a significant emphasis on economics.

There is some justification for diagnostics based entirely on curiosity as this does stimulate enthusiasm and interest that can then be channeled to the objectives of risk management. The management practices of those involved in cattle production may become quite routine, and it is often helpful to use diagnostic information as reminders of the processes that respond to better management.

DIAGNOSTIC APPROACHES

The primary and most frequently used methods of diagnosis are clinical observation and history. Complete and scientific diagnostic evaluations on every ill animal are obviously inefficient and unnecessary. The clinical approach to diagnosis must be supplemented in some cases, and judgment must be applied with regard to how extensive the effort should be. Additional methods of obtaining diagnostic information include sampling of live animals, necropsies of dead animals, and analysis of records; the latter is often a key indicator that something is wrong.

SAMPLING TECHNIQUES

Nasal swabs are frequently used in diagnostic procedures that go beyond observation and body temperature evaluation. The technique used to collect nasal swab samples is very important. The external nares should be cleaned with a dry absorbent material if badly soiled. Swabs should then be carefully inserted into the nostril, and it is generally preferred that samples be taken as deep as the swab length permits. Good restraint is necessary because the procedure is often objectionable to the animal. The purpose of swabbing must be identified before procedures begin. For instance, when taking specimens for microbial isolation, a dry swab is often utilized, which is then subsequently inserted into some type of moisture source or specific transport media to aid preservation; usually, it is best to immediately refrigerate this type of sample (there are exceptions) and rapidly convey it to a laboratory. Sampling for viruses may involve rather fragile organisms such as bovine respiratory syncytial virus (BRSV). For these types of samples, many laboratories prefer that the swab be made of Dacron™ rather than cotton, that it be inserted into a previously obtained transport medium, and that it be immediately frozen at dry ice temperatures. This allows transportation of the preparation to the laboratory in a rather stable condition.

Hematology is occasionally used as a general diagnostic technique. It probably has minimal application in differentiating the causes of BRD. Blood cultures are occasionally useful in that bacterial causes of BRD are often systemic so identification in other tissues such as blood is feasible.

Serology is a commonly used method of evaluating BRD. It can be used to profile incoming animals or to monitor infectious processes. The most important factors in obtaining serology samples are that blood should be collected in a clean tube that has not been previously used or washed and that the serum should be separated from the clot as soon as possible after blood collection. Most serologic testing can then be performed on serum that has been refrigerated for a period of several days. If samples are to be stored longer, freezing is usually not detrimental. Paired acute and convalescent serum titers may be helpful in determining recent infections.

Additional sampling opportunities include feed analyses and collection of specimens at the time of necropsy.

The most important factor in sampling techniques is communication with the testing laboratories to ensure a common understanding of methods and expectations.

Necropsy Techniques

Success or failure in evaluating BRD is often directly correlated with the number of necropsies performed either in a critical situation or as a routine. Necropsies are more easily performed by those with the appropriate equipment, and a simple necropsy kit can be very easily assembled and transported.[1] Minimal equipment includes a knife, sharpening instrument, scissors, forceps, and an axe or hatchet. Itinerant veterinarians can often rely on clients to supply all or some of this equipment. When evaluating an animal that has died and in which BRD is suspected, it is important to do an overall evaluation with regard to dehydration and body condition. It is not unusual to find evidence of severe diarrhea that has not been reported in the history. The general object of the necropsy is to classify, characterize, and, hopefully, determine the age of the lesions. Identification and characterization of lesions depend on experience and practice. It is important to develop techniques that assist in differentiating between normal tissue, abnormal tissue, and postmortem changes.

Any necropsy procedure is incomplete without a record of the observations. This can be done in any number of simple ways, usually involving abbreviated comments to maximize efficiency.

Sampling of tissues normally includes collection of fresh and formalin-fixed samples of affected and normal lung tissue, as well as tracheal samples in many cases. The fresh tissues should be at least $5 \times 5 \times 5$ cm and should be collected in a sealable, unbreakable container. Sealable plastic bags are usually the most efficient. A small insulated container should be carried to the necropsy site for best results. Formalin-fixed tissues should always be less than 1 cm in thickness and should be preserved in 10% neutral buffered formalin. It is important to augment fixation of the tissue by providing at least 10 times as much formalin solution as tissue.

Classification/Characterization of Lesions

Classification and characterization of lesions may include[2]:

- Upper respiratory disease
- Bronchial pneumonia
- Interstitial pneumonia
- Metastatic pneumonia

Upper Respiratory Disease

This generally includes observation for rhinitis (due to various causes), necrotic laryngitis, traumatic laryngitis, and tracheitis. Tracheal congestion and inflammation are often the result of terminal respiratory distress or even postmortem abdominal pressure forcing blood into the cervical region (Figure 1). These causes must be differentiated from tracheitis, which is usually the result of infection with infectious bovine rhinotracheitis (IBR) virus. Bacteri-

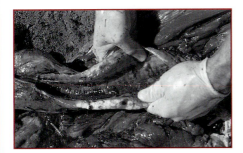

Figure 1. Congested trachea resulting from agonal breathing and postmortem abdominal pressure. There is no tracheitis.

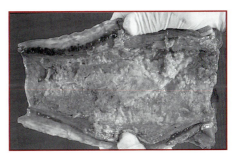

Figure 2. Diffuse fibrinous tracheitis typical of IBR.

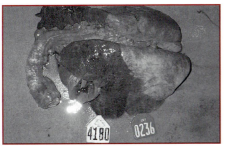

Figure 3A

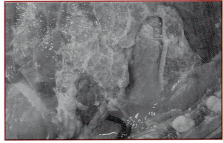

Figure 3B

Figure 3. (A) Acute pasteurellosis with fibrinous bronchial pneumonia typical of terminal stages of BRD. (B) Fibrinous pleuritis may or may not be present.

al agents may be involved, but diffuse necrotizing tracheitis is most frequently due to IBR. Careful gross evaluation allows differentiation between a discolored trachea with a smooth, shiny surface and degenerative tracheitis, where the mucosa is roughened by exudation and necrosis (Figure 2).

Bronchial Pneumonia

Bronchial pneumonias (bronchopneumonias) typical of BRD or "shipping fever" are those that are anterior and ventral in location. The lesions tend to develop through the stages of red and gray hepatization, with progression toward the upper and posterior portions of the lung. These anterior ventral lesions involve consolidation and dark discoloration.[3] It is important to understand that lesions can develop to a rather severe stage within 1 or 2 days (Figure 3). As these lesions progress, there is usually involvement of *Pasteurella haemolytica, Pasteurella multocida,* or *Haemophilus somnus.* These agents are all capable of producing associated severe pleuritis and fibrinous hydrothorax. Because of the severity of the lesions, there are often misconceptions regarding the time it takes for fulminating and fatal bronchopneumonia (Figure 4) to develop; in actuality, lesions often develop within 2 or 3 days. Lesions involving the toxin-producing microorganisms listed above often produce small necrotic foci, which then coalesce to form larger pale lesions (Figure 5). Ultimately, abscessation (Figure 6) of the areas that were initially necrotic frequently occurs.[4] This stage usually involves *Actinomyces pyogenes* and is the precursor to the undesirable "chronic" condition.

Gross evaluation can often confirm fibrinopurulent, anterior ventral pneumonia

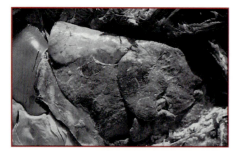

Figure 4. Acute fibrinous pneumonia caused by _H. somnus_. These lesions can develop within 2 or 3 days.

typical of BRD. There is no documented method that reliably differentiates gross pneumonic lesions produced by _P. haemolytica, P. multocida,_ or _H. somnus._ The amount of thoracic fluid and fibrin is not reliable as a differential. Some animals infected with _H. somnus_ have necrotic foci (Figure 7) in the myocardium (particularly in the papillary muscles), some have fibrinopurulent arthritis, and some may have associated thromboembolic meningoencephalitis with hemorrhages in the brain stem. However, these microorganisms frequently can be differentiated only by culture procedures.

Interstitial Pneumonia

Interstitial pneumonic lesions are typically differentiated from those of bronchial pneumonia in that they are diffusely distributed throughout the lung and are often striking, involving edema and emphysema. There may be areas of dark red discoloration and firmness interspersed with pale areas that are emphysematous. The onset of this type of pneumonia is usually quite acute and may develop within hours. Differentials that must be kept in mind include infectious agents such as BRSV, chemical agents produced in the rumen (e.g., 3–methyl indole) as a result of variation in feed intake, and, possibly, some type of allergic reactions. There are also reports of production of these lesions by mycotoxins.[3]

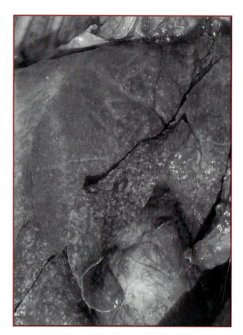

Figure 5. Lung with small necrotic foci caused by necrotizing toxins produced by _P. haemolytica_.

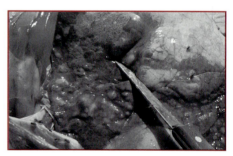

Figure 6. Chronic pneumonia with abscesses. Animals with this type of lesion may survive and often are termed "chronics."

This type of pneumonia is not usually considered to be a part of BRD, except in cases involving BRSV, which is often a copathogen in BRD.

Metastatic Pneumonia

Metastatic pneumonia is identified by multiple inflammatory foci and abscessed

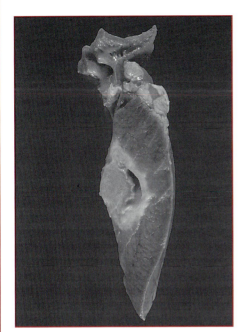

Figure 7. Heart muscle with a pale, necrotic area often observed with *H. somnus* infection. The most common location of this lesion is in the papillary muscles.

lesions scattered throughout the lungs. These findings indicate the hematogenous origin of this disease, and the initial site often involves abscesses in the liver or, possibly, wounds in another part of the body.

* * *

These general observations can be utilized for initial evaluation of general etiologic information. Laboratory assistance is often required for more specific determinations. When evaluating suspected cases of BRD, it is important to keep in mind that clinical respiratory disease may be the result of causes other than those typically associated with the BRD complex. For example, lungworms should be included in the differential list. In addition, animals with right-sided heart failure are frequently diagnosed as suffering from respiratory disease. Likewise, parasitic infections can lead to hemolysis and subse-

quent anemia, which produces signs that may be associated with respiratory disease.

LABORATORY PROCEDURES AND INTERPRETATION

Diagnosis of BRD is quite simple compared to attempts to sort out the roles of various contributing factors. Assignments of their relative significance can often be aided by laboratory support.

Bacterial cultures can help to identify a number of respiratory pathogens, including mycoplasma, chlamydia, and other bacterial agents.[5,6] Specific techniques vary between laboratories. It is always important to communicate with a laboratory beforehand so that submission of samples is suited to the techniques utilized in each individual laboratory. Communication with laboratory personnel can also assist in determining the extent of the effort (and hence the expense) to be put forth. In many cases, aerobic culture to differentiate common pathogens such as *P. haemolytica, P. multocida, H. somnus,* and *A. pyogenes* is sufficient. In other cases where the etiologies are more perplexing, it may be necessary to identify mycoplasmal and chlamydial agents. Other agents such as *Streptococcus, Staphylococcus,* and *Salmonella* spp. may also be identified. The potential importance of these agents (particularly *Salmonella* spp.) cannot be ignored. Interpretation of results is often more important than the procedures themselves. For instance, mycoplasma, chlamydia, and most of the respiratory bacteria reside in normal populations of cattle.

It is important that experience and professional judgment be applied to correlation of clinical signs, necropsy observations, and laboratory findings to determine the significance of various isolates.[7] For instance, there is evidence that *P. haemolytica* type A is normal in the upper respiratory tract but not in the pneumonic lung. Its presence in lung tissue is often associated with acute bronchopneumonia. Isolation of *P. multocida* may also be difficult to interpret. It is a frequent isolate from normal animals, it is a cause of acute bronchopneumonia, and it is often associated (more so than *P. haemolytica)* with chronic refractory pneumonias.

Sensitivity testing with regard to isolated bacteria is often a useful adjunct, but interpretation must be tempered by clinical observation. There is no absolute relationship between in vitro sensitivity and in vivo effectiveness of pharmaceutical agents. There is also no reason to believe that one or two isolates are typical of the organisms in an entire feedlot. Organisms that appear resistant to some pharmaceutical compounds in culture sometimes still respond to routine treatment of BRD. The use of sensitivity testing is often more of value for animals that are refractory to routine treatments. It can be very helpful in selecting backup medications (which are often more expensive). Sensitivity tests for *H. somnus* have not been standardized and either are not offered by many laboratories or are difficult to interpret.

Virus identification methodology has improved considerably in the past few years. Virus isolation is still the most important standard method of virus identification, but more rapid techniques such as immunochemical staining and genome identification methods are being used.[8] These permit very rapid and often highly specific identification of various viruses. Pitfalls of these techniques are based primarily on application of the information gathered. Some of these viruses are fairly frequent inhabitants of relatively normal animals so interpretation must include other information. Viruses commonly differentiated in BRD are parainfluenza-3, herpesvirus or IBR virus, BRSV, adenoviruses, rhinoviruses, and bovine viral diarrhea (BVD) virus. All of these may play some role in respiratory disease, and the various roles are often difficult to differentiate. For instance, we usually think of IBR virus as being associated with severe tracheitis, but it may also be one of the complex that helps to initiate pneumonic lesions. A serious and perplexing difficulty results from identification of BVD virus, which may play various roles in BRD. It is probably associated with

the initiation of airway lesions that lead to pneumonias. It is also extremely important in contributing to immunosuppression.

Diagnostic laboratories are frequently asked to differentiate vaccine and field strains of viruses such as IBR and BVD virus. Differentiation is always difficult and frequently impossible.

Serologic results involve considerable interpretation. Use of paired samples, including acute and convalescent periods, is extremely helpful so that increases in titers can be literally interpreted. Complicating elements include multiple vaccinations, which may induce very high titers, and numerous factors that influence antibody production. Interpretation of serology should usually be approached as a method of profiling a group of animals rather than as an absolute diagnostic test for an individual. Profiles may be helpful in establishing patterns of infection typical of certain groups of cattle or certain management situations. These can be applied in the design of control programs.

Another procedure involves evaluation of vitamin and mineral levels. It is always wise to obtain liver samples that can be refrigerated or frozen at the time of necropsy, which can be submitted for later testing to determine the possible role of nutritional inadequacies in the pathogenesis of BRD. This type of evaluation does leave some questions because it cannot be definitively known whether deficiencies are a cause of BRD or whether they are the result of illness and metabolic debilitation just before death.

Histopathology of representative areas of lung, trachea, visceral organs, and other abdominal tissues is very useful as a general method of correlating clinical signs, gross observations, and laboratory findings. Some lesions are fairly specific and can be used to answer certain questions. Often histopathology can determine whether the laboratory findings correlate with the gross observations. Diseases such as IBR, BRSV, and atypical interstitial pneumonia are subject to fairly definitive diagnosis with histopathology. Other conditions such as bacterial pneumonia most often require correlation with laboratory results.

APPLICATION OF DIAGNOSTIC INFORMATION

Diagnostic information is of no value if it has no application. In some cases, the information can be applied in immediate problem-solving measures, such as changes in prevention and treatment programs based on specific disease or etiologic identification. More frequently, the information can be used in adjusting programs and teaching production personnel better methods of health management. For instance, in a case involving extensive anterior ventral pneumonia, some small or coalescing necrotic lesions may be found in the lung. If the animal was only recently observed as ill, the conclusion must be that responsible personnel failed in *early* detection. If the animal has been treated for several days, a discussion of therapeutic efficacy may be initiated. Some lungs may have evidence of progression of lesions, including more recent lesions in the middle to upper areas. These lesions may be the result of poor treatment response or, in many cases, a failure to administer medication for an adequate length of time.

Immunization programs can also be adjusted as a result of determination of causes of losses or presence of specific disease agents.

Necropsy information should include assessment of injection sites as a means of evaluating and enhancing quality assurance programs.

SUMMARY

Diagnosis of BRD is quite easy because of characteristic history, clinical signs, and lesions. It is much more difficult to assign relative significance to many contributing factors or causes. All cases involve some type of mixed infections. The multifactorial complex of viruses, bacteria, mycoplasma, and environmental factors often precludes specific assignment of relative importance or degree of interaction.

Frequent experiences with necropsy and laboratory diagnostic procedures correlated with response to various immunization and treatment procedures should help to produce more definitive concepts of cause and effect. For instance, *Pasteurella* spp. are the obvious cause of *Pasteurella* pneumonia and death in most fatal cases of BRD. However, veterinarians throughout much of the United States are reporting increasing losses due to *H. somnus*.

Considerable judgment and personal bias still enter into interpretation of the relative importance of various environmental factors and etiologic agents. This will provide material for considerable discussion of diagnostics for the foreseeable future.

REFERENCES

1. Wren G: Getting the most out of feedlot pathology. *Bovine Vet,* pp 4–7, May 1994.
2. Pierson RE, Kainer RA: Clinical classification of pneumonias in cattle. *Bovine Pract* 15:73–76, 1980.
3. Dungworth DL: The respiratory system, in Jubb KVF, Kennedy PC, Palmer N (eds): *Pathology of Domestic Animals,* ed 4, vol 2. New York, Academic Press, 1991, pp 539–699.
4. Thompson RG: The pathogenesis and lesions of pneumonia in cattle. *Compend Contin Educ Pract Vet* 3(11):S403–S413, 1981.
5. Welsh RD: Bacterial and mycoplasma species isolated from pneumonic bovine lungs. *Agri-Practice* 14(7):12–16, 1993.
6. Breeze R: Respiratory disease in adult cattle. *Food Anim Pract* 1(2):311–345, 1985.
7. Dyer RM: The bovine respiratory disease complex: Infectious agents. *Compend Contin Educ Pract Vet* 3(10):S374–S382, 1981.
8. Jackwood MW: Biotechnology and the development of diagnostic tests in veterinary medicine. *JAVMA* 204(10):1603–1605, 1994.

Significance of Bacterial Culture and Sensitivities in Bovine Respiratory Disease

Cyril R. Clarke, BVSc, PhD, Associate Professor
Diplomate ACVCP
Department of Physiological Science
College of Veterinary Medicine
Oklahoma State University
Stillwater, Oklahoma

In vitro antibacterial sensitivity assays, such as the agar disk diffusion technique and direct determination of minimum inhibitory concentrations (MICs), can be used to guide selection of antibacterial agents for therapy of bovine respiratory disease (BRD). Caution should be exercised in interpreting such data, however, as they are generally derived from assays that do not take into account conditions that occur in vivo, such as the contribution of host defenses to antibacterial efficacy or the effect of inflammatory responses on activity of antibacterial agents. Furthermore, the predictive value of in vitro sensitivity data depends on the origin and relevance of the bacterial isolate subjected to culture and sensitivity testing. Nevertheless, when used appropriately, in vitro sensitivity testing constitutes an important stage in the development of efficacious therapeutic protocols. Rational interpretation of in vitro antibacterial sensitivity results requires a thorough understanding of the relevance of isolates collected from different sites in the respiratory tract, the clinical status of the animal from which samples are collected, the methodology used to conduct various types of in vitro sensitivity assays, the assumptions associated with each method, and the relationship between culture and sensitivity determinations and pharmacokinetic disposition.

ISOLATION OF BACTERIA FOR CULTURE AND SENSITIVITY ASSAY

Identification of Relevant Bacterial Isolates

Ideally, samples collected for culture and sensitivity testing should contain the primary etiologic pathogen and should not be contaminated with inconsequential isolates. Furthermore, samples should be collected, preserved, packaged, and transported in such a manner that the viability of the microorganisms is maintained. These requirements are sometimes difficult to satisfy in the managerial and physical environment in which feedlot or stocker cattle are maintained.

Pasteurella haemolytica, the organism most frequently isolated from the lungs of feedlot cattle with bacterial pneumonia, is considered to be the most common and important causative agent of BRD. The involvement of *P. haemolytica* in a majority of cases implies that an isolate collected from a single animal is representative of the pneumonia-causing bacteria in other animals. Unfortunately, this assumption is not valid because the microbiology of BRD may be extremely complex. In addition to *P. haemolytica,* other microorganisms such as *Pasteurella multocida, Mycoplasma* spp., *Pseudomonas aeruginosa, Haemophilus somnus,* and *Actinomyces pyogenes* have also been implicated as etiologic agents of BRD.[1-6] Even in animals that are experimentally infected with pure cultures of *P. haemolytica, P. multocida* has been isolated from the lung after inoculation.[a] An argument can be made that these microorganisms are unlikely to be primary etiologic agents and therefore can be ignored in the formulation of therapeutic protocols. Although this argument may be valid when

[a]Clarke CR: Unpublished data.

selecting primary antibacterial agents for initial use against outbreaks of BRD, all isolates must be considered when animals do not respond to initial treatment and secondary antibacterial agents are to be selected. This is especially important in cases of subacute or chronic pneumonia, when the initial etiologic agent may no longer be the predominant infecting microorganism. Indeed, an assumption that *P. haemolytica* is the only important causative organism in a particular feedlot or stocker calf operation may lead to inappropriate drug selection and high treatment failure rates. Therefore in vitro sensitivity data pertinent to all relevant isolates should be evaluated when antibacterial treatment protocols are developed.

Aside from the involvement of a diversity of microbial species, pneumonia caused by *P. haemolytica* alone may not be homogeneous. *P. haemolytica* type A consists of several different serotypes that may themselves be divided into many strains. Recently, the application of molecular genetic techniques has confirmed that the microbiology of BRD is extremely complex.[7] Using ribotyping and restriction endonuclease analysis, strains of *P. haemolytica* involved in a single outbreak of BRD have been shown to vary between animals and even within a single animal. Unfortunately, antibacterial sensitivities of specific strains of *P. haemolytica* may vary considerably. Thus the antibacterial sensitivity of *P. haemolytica* for most antimicrobial agents is unpredictable, requiring that treatment strategies be matched to in vitro sensitivities of each relevant etiologic isolate.

Obviously, culture and sensitivity testing cannot be performed on every individual animal diagnosed with BRD. Managerial and economic constraints, coupled with the necessity of treating pneumonic animals as soon as possible, would prohibit such a strategy. On the other hand, the heterogeneous population of microorganisms involved in BRD precludes basing selection of antimicrobial therapy for an entire feedlot or stocker operation use on culture and sensitivity results from samples from a single animal. Therefore it is recommended that a large number of random culture and sensitivity tests be performed (and the database be updated accordingly) at least twice a year, for example, during the fall and the winter, when most outbreaks of BRD occur. Alternatively, animals could be sampled at the start of an outbreak of BRD and then again when resistant populations of bacteria have emerged. Depending on the geographic origin of cattle shipped to a feedlot, specific pens or groups of pens may need to be tested to obtain relevant data. These data should only be applied to the appropriate reference population.

Collection of Microbiologic Samples

Samples for culture and sensitivity testing are usually collected from the nasal cavity, the laryngotracheal region, or the lung. Great care should be exercised to ensure that samples contain relevant pathogens and are not contaminated with inconsequential microorganisms. Swabs must not come into contact with any surfaces other than relevant nasopharyngeal or respiratory mucosa, and lavage buffers must be directly delivered to and collected from the region of interest. Nasal swabs must be inserted through the nostril for collection of samples from the nasal cavity; samples of nasal discharge from the exterior of the muzzle are likely to be contaminated with other microorganisms that overgrow the offending pathogen when cultured. These contaminants may suppress the growth of the etiologic bacterium or can so confuse diagnosis that additional time-consuming isolations become necessary. Contaminants present a particular problem when the offending pathogen grows fastidiously on diagnostic media.

Laryngotracheal samples are best collected using equine uterine swabs. The animal should be restrained using a head gate and nose tongs; the dorsum of the tongue is then depressed, and the laryngeal folds are illuminated while the swab is inserted into the trachea.

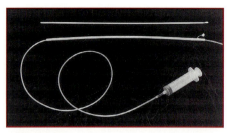

Figure 1A

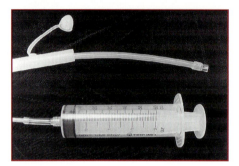

Figure 1B
Figure 1. Equipment that may be used to conduct lung lavage. Once a guarded equine uterine catheter (A) **(Kallaja Industries, Inc., Long Beach, CA) has been inserted into the trachea, the swab is removed and a flexible plastic tube connected to a syringe is threaded through the catheter sleeve** (B) **into the lung.**

Lung lavage is accomplished in a similar fashion. A flexible plastic tube approximately 4 feet in length is passed through the outer sleeve of an equine uterine catheter after it has been positioned in the trachea and the swab has been removed (Figure 1). When the flexible catheter cannot be threaded any further into the distal airways, 50 ml of sterile buffer is injected and then immediately aspirated.

The two most important considerations in shipping samples for microbiologic isolation are prevention of desiccation and refrigeration. Desiccation is most likely to occur when nasal or laryngotracheal swabs are stored or transported without media. Culturette-type swabs that contain prepackaged media provide a convenient means of avoiding desiccation and contamination. Refrigeration is best achieved by packing samples in Styrofoam-insulated, leakproof containers with refrigerant packs. Appropriately packaged samples must be analyzed as soon as possible after collection and therefore should be hand delivered or sent via overnight courier service to the diagnostic laboratory.

P. haemolytica is a normal inhabitant of the nasal mucosa of healthy cattle; when host defense mechanisms are compromised by physical stress or viral infection, however, the bacterium undergoes very rapid multiplication. Bacteria-laden aerosol droplets are then inhaled into the lung, causing acute fibrinopurulent pneumonia.[8,9] In light of the fact that the pathogenesis of shipping fever pneumonia involves all components of the respiratory system, samples collected from any anatomic region of the respiratory tract should be suitable for isolation of the etiologic microorganism. Thus collection of samples from the nasal mucosa should yield isolates that are representative of those colonizing the lung. However, although *P. haemolytica* is a normal inhabitant of bovine nasal mucosa, the serotypes colonizing this site are not necessarily those responsible for pneumonia. In comparison with diseased animals, healthy animals have a higher ratio of *P. haemolytica* serotype 2 to serotype 1 isolations.[10] Serotype 1 biotype A is usually implicated in pneumonic pasteurellosis. Therefore the in vitro antibacterial sensitivities of isolates cultured from the nasal cavity of healthy cattle may not be predictive of those involved in an outbreak of pneumonia. This is unfortunate because it precludes screening of cattle when they are initially processed on arrival at the feedlot. Even when animals are stressed and *P. haemolytica* serotype 1 has overgrown other serotypes and bacteria in the nasopharyngeal region, nasal swab samples may not adequately represent bacteria colonizing the lung. In several experiments, antimicrobial susceptibilities of *P. haemolytica* isolated from the upper respiratory tract have been found to be different from those of the lower respiratory tract. In one study, for example, nasopharyngeal isolates had a higher incidence of resistance to penicillin G, ampicillin, and oxytetracycline than did those isolated from pneumonic lungs.[11]

Therefore lung lavage samples are collected from the most relevant tissue region; when collected aseptically, these samples are least likely to contain inconsequential contaminants. Although lung lavage is easily accomplished with trained personnel and suitable cattle handling facilities, it is not a practical option in the feedlot environment because it is time consuming and subject to many methodologic errors. Collection of nasal samples is most easily achieved, but the results are the least reliable because of the accessibility of this region to contaminants. Laryngotracheal swabs, which offer a balance between ease of collection and relevance of results, are therefore recommended.

Clinical Status of Animals

Ideally, samples for antibacterial sensitivity testing should be collected from pneumonic animals prior to treatment. As stated previously, the antibacterial sensitivities of pathogenic *P. haemolytica* involved in BRD may be different from those of bacteria residing in the nasal cavity prior to infection. Also, selection of antibacterial agents based solely on culture and sensitivity testing of samples collected from dead animals should be avoided. The antibacterial sensitivities of pathogens isolated from these treatment failures are unlikely to be representative of pathogens infecting most cattle in the feedlot. Similarly, although samples collected from live animals that have not responded satisfactorily to antibacterial therapy may provide useful information concerning the identity and antibacterial susceptibilities of pathogens infecting those particular animals, they are probably not representative of the pathogenic bacterial population as a whole. Not only does the incidence of bacterial resistance to a particular antibacterial agent increase when animals have received that agent, but resistance to other antibacterial agents is increased as well.[3] Therefore periodic sampling of animals diagnosed with BRD but not yet treated with antibacterial agents should be used to select antibacterial agents for initial therapy; data derived from subsequent testing of antibacterial-treated animals can be used to identify suitable agents for treating those animals that do not respond to initial therapy.

TYPES OF IN VITRO SENSITIVITY TESTS

Laboratory Techniques

The most commonly used method of measuring in vitro antibacterial sensitivity is the agar disk diffusion technique. Interpretation of results depends on the size of a zone of inhibition produced when Mueller-Hinton agar is inoculated for confluent growth of a bacterial isolate and then incubated in the presence of a filter paper disk impregnated with a standard concentration of antibacterial agent. As the antibacterial agent diffuses out through the media, the concentration of antibacterial agent in the agar decreases as the distance from the paper disk increases. The edge of the zone of inhibition is the point at which antibacterial concentrations are low enough to allow bacterial growth; the concentration at this point is similar to the MIC. Obviously, an isolate that is very sensitive to an antibacterial agent will have a low MIC and a large zone of inhibition. Based on reference scattergrams consisting of zones of inhibition plotted against MICs of a large number of isolates, interpretative zone standards of susceptible, resistant, or intermediate (moderately susceptible) are established by selecting MIC breakpoints.[12] The MIC breakpoint is the concentration of an antibacterial agent that must be exceeded to achieve optimal therapy. Selection of the MIC breakpoint is based on the pharmacokinetic disposition of approved doses, the population distribution of MICs for isolates with comparable susceptibilities, and documented clinical responses of isolates to approved doses. The clinical interpretation of zone standards is as follows[13]:

- Isolates classified as *susceptible* are expected to be inhibited by concentrations of antibacterial agent attained in the blood following administration of approved doses.
- Isolates classified as *resistant* are not expected to be affected by administration of approved doses.
- Isolates classified as *intermediate* are considered to be susceptible only when maximum recommended/tolerated doses are administered. Generally, selection of antibacterial agents for use against microorganisms with intermediate susceptibility classifications is discouraged.

Another common approach to estimate in vitro antibacterial susceptibility is direct measurement of MICs. In this method a standard inoculum of a bacterial isolate is incubated with serial dilutions of antibacterial agent. The lowest concentration of antibacterial agent that inhibits growth is defined as the MIC. Recent use of microtitration trays containing dehydrated antibacterial agents has greatly facilitated routine MIC determination and the availability of MIC data.[14,15] Results may be reported as original MIC data or in terms of susceptibility classifications using breakpoints, as described above.

Assumptions and Limitations

The common use by veterinary diagnostic laboratories of commercial microtitration trays formulated for human pathogens often presents problems. This is particularly true when MICs against *P. haemolytica* are determined because the bacterial sensitivity spectrum of this bacterium is unusual. For example, macrolides (erythromycin, tylosin, tilmicosin) are usually considered to be effective primarily against gram-positive bacteria and, consequently, are not usually included on commercial microtitration trays containing media appropriate for culture of gram-negative bacteria. Obviously, evaluation of culture and sensitivity data pertinent to macrolides is essential when antibacterial

treatment strategies against BRD are developed. Furthermore, all of the antibacterial agents approved or recommended for use against BRD may not be included in these commercial trays. Usually, predictions have to be made based on sensitivity to antibacterial agents in the same chemical group. For example, ceftazidime, ciprofloxacin, sulfamethoxazole, tetracycline, and chloramphenicol can be used to represent ceftiofur, enrofloxacin, sulfachlorpyridazine, oxytetracycline, and florfenicol, respectively. Unfortunately, this approach may not always be reliable because some chemical groups of antibacterial agents, such as the sulfonamides, can vary considerably with regard to their spectrum of activity. Furthermore, use of chloramphenicol instead of florfenicol is likely to result in underestimation of sensitivity to florfenicol.[16] The alternative is to order custom formulated trays appropriate for veterinary pathogens, but these are often expensive.

Both the agar disk diffusion assay and direct determination of MIC are conducted in the absence of host defense and inflammatory responses and therefore may not be predictive of in vivo efficacy.[17] Antibacterial agents that usually achieve bacteriostatic rather than bactericidal concentrations in sites of infection merely inhibit bacterial growth and rely on immune mechanisms to eradicate the infection. Thus in vitro susceptibility may underestimate in vivo efficacy of these agents. Conversely, antibacterial agents judged to be effective in vitro may be inactivated in the animal by cultural conditions resulting from inflammatory processes and tissue damage. Conditions responsible for antibacterial inactivation include binding of drug to plasma and acute phase proteins (e.g., albumin and α1-acid glycoprotein), changes in pH that alter the diffusion of drug into infected tissues and bacteria, and accumulation of cellular debris, which may serve as a source of metabolic intermediates that negate the mechanism of action of the drug.

One of the criteria used to classify bacterial isolates as being susceptible, resistant, or intermediate is that the breakpoint concentration must be lower than the concentration of antibacterial agent attainable in the blood following administration of an approved dose. This assumes that there is a direct correlation between blood concentration and in vivo efficacy. However, in vivo efficacy is related to the concentration of drug at the site of action in the lung, and pulmonary tissue concentrations may be substantially higher or lower than corresponding blood concentrations, depending on the lipid solubility of the antibacterial agent. For example, erythromycin,[18] tilmicosin,[b] and danofloxacin[19] accumulate within lung tissue, where concentrations may be 3 to 15 times greater than corresponding serum concentrations. In contrast to the macrolides and fluoroquinolones, aminoglycosides and β-lactams penetrate lung tissue poorly, with the result that lung concentrations are usually only 25% to 30% of corresponding serum concentrations.[20] Aside from the extent of tissue distribution, the concentration-time profile observed in tissues may be quite different from that occurring in blood.[17] With the exception of macrolides, fluoroquinolones, and trimethoprim, peak concentrations in tissues are lower and are achieved later than corresponding blood peak concentrations. Furthermore, the rate of drug elimination from tissues is lower than from blood, resulting in more prolonged tissue concentrations. Differences between dispositional profiles in blood and lung tissue are even more marked in cases of subacute or chronic pneumonia, because abscessation and consolidation of lung tissue present barriers to drug diffusion. Drug concentrations in bronchial secretions, as opposed to lung tissue, correlate more closely with those in blood[21,22] and are probably of predictive value only during the early acute phase of pneumonia, prior to accumulation of fibropurulent exudate and development of diffusional barriers.

Considering that susceptibility classifications (susceptible, resistant, or intermediate) are determined using MIC breakpoints based on blood concentrations that do not correlate well with lung tissue concentrations and that the breakpoints customarily used by veterinary laboratories are estimated from human pharmacokinetic data and approved doses rather than those appropriate for cattle, use of these classifications is discouraged. Indeed, there is little difference between susceptibility classifications based on disk diffusion assays or direct determination of MICs because in both cases interpretation is subject to the same flawed process governing selection of MIC breakpoints. Until reliable breakpoints are established for cattle, it is recommended that susceptibility classifications not be used; rather, original MICs should be used in conjunction with pharmacokinetic data describing disposition of antibacterial agents in cattle. This would provide a more quantitative approach that is more likely to result in satisfactory treatment responses.

SELECTION OF ANTIBACTERIAL AGENTS BASED ON MICS AND PHARMACOKINETIC DISPOSITION

The primary goal of antibacterial therapy is to achieve an effective concentration of drug at the site of infection for a duration sufficient to cause elimination of bacteria. To achieve this goal, antibacterial agents that are selected for use against BRD should attain concentrations in infected lung tissue that exceed the MIC established in vitro. Ideally, this requirement should be satisfied after administration of the approved labeled dose, thus avoiding toxicity and food residue concerns. An essential requirement necessary to this approach is accurate pharmacokinetic data describing disposition of antibacterial agents in infected lung tissue. Although numerous mathematic equations can be used to calculate specific dosage regimens that can achieve satisfactory tissue concentrations,[23] these are complex and are probably not of practical use in the feedlot environment. Consequently, therapy can be guided by correlating MIC values with predicted serum

[b]Product information, Elanco Animal Health.

TABLE 1

Maximum Serum Concentrations, Minimum Serum Concentrations at the End of Dosage Intervals, Degree of Penetration into Lung Tissue, and Estimated Peak Lung Concentrations Likely to Be Achieved after Administration of a Single Approved or Recommended Dose of Antibacterial Agents

Drug	Approved/ Recommended Dosage (Interval)	C_{max}^a (µg/ml)	C_{min}^a (µg/ml)	% Penetration	L_{max} (µg/ml)
Penicillin G	Penicillin G procaine + penicillin G benzathine: 8818 IU/kg SC (48 hr)	0.59	0.01	25	0.15
	Penicillin G procaine: 6614 IU/kg IM (24 hr)	0.62	0.03	25	0.16
Ampicillin	4.4–11 mg/kg IM (24 hr)	9.40	1.60	25	2.35
Amoxicillin	6.6–11 mg/kg SC, IM (24 hr)	5.19	1.36	25	1.30
Ceftiofur	1–2 mg/kg IM (24 hr)	4.58	0.05	30[b]	1.37
Erythromycin	15 mg/kg IM (24 hr)[c]	2.4	0.15	250	6.00
Lincomycin	11 mg/kg IM (24 hr)[c]	7.17	0.06	50	3.60
Oxytetracycline	6.6–11 mg/kg IV, IM (24 hr)				
	Hydrochloride	4.37	1.17	65	2.84
	Base	2.93	1.30	65	1.91
Florfenicol	20 mg/kg IM (48 hr)[e]	3.07	0.57[d]	100	3.07
Spectinomycin	20 mg/kg IM (12 hr)[c]	52.54	0.05	30	15.76
Sulfachlorpyridazine	40 mg/kg IV (12 hr)	166.71[e]	0.13	—	—
Sulfadimethoxine	55 mg/kg IV, then 27.5 mg/kg IV (24 hr)	297.30[e]	34.25	50	148.65
Sulfadiazine	17.6 mg/kg IV (24 hr)[c,f]	20.65[e]	0.12	—	—
Tilmicosin	10 mg/kg SC (1 dose only)	0.64	—	1450	9.28
Trimethoprim	3.5 mg/kg IV (24 hr)[c]	1.78[e]	0.01	300	5.34
Tylosin	17.6 mg/kg IM (12 hr)	1.85	0.42	500	9.24

Table adapted from Clarke and associates[17] and updated to include tilmicosin (product information, Elanco Animal Health) and florfenicol.[24,25]

C_{max} = maximum serum concentration; C_{min} = minimum serum concentration at the end of the dosage interval; % penetration = degree of penetration; L_{max} = peak concentration achieved in the lung = (C_{max} × % penetration).

[a]Using highest approved/recommended dose and dosage interval.

[b]May be 50%–60% in *P. haemolytica*–infected tissue (Clarke and coworkers, unpublished data).

[c]Not approved for use in all countries. Check with your local regulatory authority.

[d]Value estimated using pharmacokinetic data in Lobell and coworkers.[24]

[e]Zero time plasma concentration.

[f]Combined with trimethoprim.

concentrations and the degree of penetration into lung tissue. It is the author's opinion that the minimum requirement for use of a specific antibacterial agent is that the peak concentration achieved in the lung (L_{max}) should at least exceed the MIC. The L_{max} may be estimated using the degree of penetration (% penetration),[17] which is expressed as a proportion of the maximum serum concentration (C_{max}; see Table 1).[17,24,25] For example, if an isolate has an MIC for erythromycin of 4 μg/ml, administration of a recommended dose[26] (15 mg/kg) will probably result in a favorable response because the L_{max} (C_{max} × % penetration = 2.4 μg/ml × 250% = 6 μg/ml) exceeds MIC. Thus erythromycin is expected to accumulate within lung tissue such that concentrations exceeding the MIC will be achieved. If one were to consider only the C_{max}, which is considerably lower than the MIC, selection of erythromycin would not be well justified. Intermittent dosing of bactericidal agents (penicillins, aminoglycosides), which results in plasma concentrations that exceed MIC for only part of the dosage interval, appears to be as efficacious as maintaining concentrations above MIC.[27] Depending on the potential for toxicity and regulatory restrictions, exceeding the labeled dose may be appropriate when the approved dose is not likely to achieve satisfactory lung concentrations and there are no alternative approved drugs. Appropriate higher doses may be estimated using relevant MICs and dosage calculation equations described elsewhere.[17,23]

SUMMARY

The following guidelines governing collection of microbiologic samples and use of in vitro sensitivity testing are recommended:

- Several times a year a large number of random samples should be collected from animals diagnosed with BRD but not yet treated with antibacterial agents. Culture and sensitivity data derived from these animals can be used to identify agents suitable for initial therapy.

Data derived from subsequent testing of treatment failures can be used to guide selection of agents for those animals not responding to initial therapy.

- Samples for isolation of pathogenic microorganisms should be collected from the laryngotracheal region. Samples should be refrigerated and desiccation should be avoided.

- Culture and sensitivity data used to formulate antibacterial selection priorities should be updated at least twice a year and considered relevant only for the reference population.

- Until more reliable breakpoints relevant to veterinary medicine are universally available, use of susceptibility classifications should be avoided. Instead, original MIC data should be used to select an antibacterial agent that can at least achieve an estimated peak lung concentration that exceeds the MIC.

- Doses that exceed the labeled dose may be necessary. These can be calculated using appropriate pharmacokinetic equations, but the veterinarian must remain aware of regulatory restrictions and the potential for toxicity.

REFERENCES

1. Hjerpe CA, Rouen TA: Practical and theoretical considerations concerning treatment of bacterial pneumonia in feedlot cattle, with special reference to antimicrobic therapy. *Proc AABP* 9:97, 1976.
2. Jensen R, Pierson RE, Braddy PM, et al: Shipping fever pneumonia in yearling feedlot cattle. *JAVMA* 169:500, 1976.
3. Martin SW, Meek AH, Curtis RA: Antimicrobial use in feedlot calves: Its association with culture rates and antimicrobial susceptibility. *Can J Comp Med* 47:6, 1983.
4. Van Amstel SR, Henton M, Witcomb MA, et al: Antibiotic sensitivity of *Pasteurella haemolytica* isolated by means of a fibreoptic endoscope from cases of pneumonic pasteurellosis in cattle. *Onderstepoort J Vet Res* 54:551, 1987.
5. Welsh RD: Seasonal incidence of bovine respiratory bacterial pathogens—OADDL (1992). Report of the Oklahoma Animal Disease Diagnostic Laboratory, 1993.
6. Welsh RD: Bacterial and mycoplasma species isolated from pneumonic bovine lungs. *Agri-*

Practice 14(7):14, 1993.

7. Murphy GL, Robinson LC, Burrows GE: Restriction endonuclease analysis and ribotyping differentiate *Pasteurella haemolytica* serotype A1 isolates from cattle within a feedlot. *J Clin Microbiol* 31(9):2303, 1993.

8. Wilkie BN, Shewen P: Defining the role that *Pasteurella haemolytica* plays in shipping fever. *Vet Med* 83:105, 1988.

9. Frank GH: When *Pasteurella haemolytica* colonizes the nasal passages of cattle. *Vet Med* 83:1060, 1988.

10. Wray C, Thompson DA: Serotypes of *Pasteurella haemolytica* isolated from calves. *Br Vet J* 127:66, 1971.

11. Allan EM, Gibbs HA, Shoo MK, et al: Antimicrobial sensitivities of *Pasteurella haemolytica* A1 from beef calves. *Vet Rec* 117:629, 1985.

12. Acar JF, Goldstein FW: Disk susceptibility test, in Lorian V (ed): *Antibiotics in Laboratory Medicine*. Baltimore, Williams & Wilkins, 1986, p 27.

13. Welsh RD: MIC antimicrobial testing and combination antibiotics. *Texas Vet Med Diag Lab Rep* 38(2):17, 1987.

14. Phillips I, Warren C, Waterworth PM: Determination of antibiotic sensitivities by the Sensititre system. *J Clin Pathol* 31:531, 1978.

15. Fales WH, Burrows GE: A new in vitro susceptibility testing system for veterinary medical diagnostic laboratories using a commercially prepared stabilized and dried antimicrobial minimal inhibitory concentration system. *Proc Am Assoc Vet Lab Diagn* 26:77, 1983.

16. Lockwood PW, de Haas V, Katz T, Varma KJ: Clinical efficacy of florfenicol in the treatment of bovine respiratory disease in North America. Proceedings of an International Symposium on Bovine Respiratory Disease—New Therapeutic Advances, held in association with the XVIII World Buiatrics Congress, Bologna, 1994, p 31.

17. Clarke CR, Burrows GE, Ames TR: Therapy of bovine bacterial pneumonia. *Vet Clin North Am Food Anim Pract* 7:669, 1991.

18. Burrows GE: Effects of experimentally induced *Pasteurella haemolytica* pneumonia on the pharmacokinetics of erythromycin in the calf. *Am J Vet Res* 46(4):798, 1985.

19. Apley MD, Upson DW: Lung tissue concentrations and plasma pharmacokinetics of danofloxacin in calves with acute pneumonia. *Am J Vet Res* 54:937, 1993.

20. Burrows GE: Systematic antibacterial drug selection and dosage. *Bovine Pract* 15:103, 1980.

21. Friis C: Penetration of danofloxacin into the respiratory tract tissues and secretions in calves. *Am J Vet Res* 54(7):1122, 1993.

22. Halstead SL, Walker RD, Baker JC, et al: Pharmacokinetic evaluation of ceftiofur in serum, tissue chamber fluid and bronchial secretions from healthy beef-bred calves. *Can J Vet Res* 56(4):269, 1992.

23. Gibaldi M, Perrier D: One-compartment model, in *Pharmacokinetics*. New York, Marcel Dekker, 1975, p 1.

24. Lobell RD, Varma KJ, Johnson JC, et al: Pharmacokinetics of florfenicol following intravenous and intramuscular doses to cattle. *J Vet Pharmacol Therap* 17:253, 1994.

25. Adams PE, Varma KJ, Powers TE, Lamendola JF: Tissue concentrations and pharmacokinetics of florfenicol in male veal calves given repeated doses. *Am J Vet Res* 48:1725, 1987.

26. Burrows GE, Griffin DD, Pippin A, Harris K: A comparison of the various routes of administration of erythromycin in cattle. *J Vet Pharmacol Ther* 12:289, 1989.

27. Koritz GD: Relevance of peak and trough concentrations to antimicrobial therapy. *JAVMA* 185:1072, 1984.

Therapeutic Management of the Bovine Respiratory Disease Complex

Robert A. Smith, DVM, MS, McCasland Chair in
Beef Health and Production
Diplomate ABVP
Boren Veterinary Medical Teaching Hospital
Oklahoma State University
Stillwater, Oklahoma

Treatment of the bovine respiratory disease complex (BRDC) is an important part of health management programs for stocker and feeder cattle. The basic goal of health management programs should be to minimize disease; however, calves continue to develop and require treatment for bovine respiratory disease (BRD). It is impossible to eliminate all cases of BRDC, even given today's management and technology. In 1968, Dr. George L. Crenshaw said, "Respiratory diseases of cattle, particularly those associated with shipping fever, are extremely complex, and it is questionable that they will ever be solved completely with our present methods of weaning, processing, shipping and handling after arrival at the feedlot."[1] For the most part, this statement is still true today.

BRDC refers to shipping fever pneumonia, more accurately described as fibrinous pneumonia and bronchopneumonia. This disease complex is the primary focus of this article. This is not intended to minimize the importance of other lower respiratory tract diseases (e.g., atypical interstitial pneumonia, metastatic pneumonia, verminous pneumonia or fibrinous pleuritis and pleuropneumonia), but these conditions have a more sporadic impact. Upper respiratory diseases such as diphtheria, tracheal edema, laryngeal abscesses, and rhinitis are also important in stocker and feeder cattle. Nevertheless, BRDC is by far the most important respiratory disease challenging the industry.[2,3]

TREATMENT PROGRAM OBJECTIVES

The treatment program plays an impor-tant role in minimizing losses due to respiratory disease. Objectives of the treatment program include:

- Reduction of death loss
- Reduction in the rate of chronic cases
- Improvement of performance in calves that have been sick
- Improvement of animal welfare
- Cost effectiveness

EVALUATION OF THE SICK CALF

Personnel responsible for treatment of sick cattle should evaluate the calves once the animals are in the hospital area. This allows confirmation of the diagnosis made by the pencheckers (penriders) and increases familiarity with the presenting clinical signs. The most prominent clinical signs are depression and inappetence, which is manifested by a gaunt appearance. Dyspnea is not common in acute cases of bovine respiratory disease,[4,5] but respiration rate may be increased if the body temperature is elevated, the ambient temperature is high, or the calf has been physically stressed during movement to the hospital area. Paroxysmal coughing is not common although a soft, moist cough may be elicited by exercise. Nasal and ocular discharges are often present but do not correlate well with the severity of disease.

The rectal temperature of calves with BRD ranges from 103.5° to 108° F. Many feedlot practitioners initiate antibiotic therapy when rectal temperature is 104° F or higher, although the exact critical rectal temperature has not been scientifically determined. It is useful to assign and record "severity of illness" or "degree of illness" scores (0 = healthy, 1 = slightly ill, 2 = moderately ill, 3 = severely ill, 4 = moribund) to provide a subjective method of monitoring treatment response. This is particularly helpful when large numbers of cattle are undergoing treatment as individuals tend to lose identity.

ANTIBIOTIC SELECTION

The selection of the proper antibiotic regimen for treatment of BRD is an important part of the treatment program. Four methods are commonly used to select antibiotics:

- Antemortem testing
- Postmortem testing
- Literature (field trials)
- Evaluation of clinical response

Culture and antibiotic sensitivity testing has long been used by practitioners as a guide for selection of antibiotics for treatment of BRD. Historically, the samples submitted to the laboratory have been obtained at necropsy, and results from such testing can be misleading. *Pasteurella* spp. isolated from calves treated with antimicrobials tend to demonstrate increased resistance to those same antimicrobials.[6,7] Some degree of cross-resistance to other antibiotics also occurs. This strongly suggests that the best antibiotic sensitivity test results are obtained from antemortem samples from untreated, febrile calves showing typical signs of BRD.

Two in vitro susceptibility tests are commonly used: (1) the Kirby-Bauer disk diffusion or culture sensitivity test, and (2) determination of minimum inhibitory concentrations (MICs). The culture sensitivity test is based on antimicrobial drug concentrations in the blood of humans and the susceptibility pattern of populations of fast growing aerobic bacteria. It is qualitative in nature and overestimates susceptibility of bacteria in sites where blood perfusion is poor and underestimates bacterial susceptibility in tissues where drugs concentrate

physiologically.[8] The usefulness of the culture sensitivity test for selecting appropriate antimicrobials for treatment of BRD is highly suspect.[9–11] MIC data allow the veterinarian to utilize pharmacokinetic information more effectively, but MIC results still have limitations. These results do not consider the extent of tissue involvement, contribution of host defenses, virulence of the organism, or effect of subinhibitory doses of antibiotics on bacterial susceptibility.[8,9] Overall there is a poor correlation between the MIC and the fatality rate due to *Pasteurella haemolytica*.[9] Until more information is available, MIC results from large populations of untreated calves can serve as a guide to antibiotic selection and dosage. They should not, however, be considered the final authority for selecting or rejecting a particular antimicrobial.

Necropsy, or postmortem, examination of calves serves to confirm the clinical diagnosis and often can help explain perceived or actual treatment failures. In many fatal cases of BRD, concomitant diseases or conditions (e.g., viral infections, enteric disease, and injuries) limit success of antimicrobial treatment. A thorough history of the dead calf and its penmates helps to correlate pneumonic lesions with arrival time, treatment days, and therapy used. As previously discussed, submission of samples from treated calves for in vitro sensitivity testing is likely to be of no value.

Published field trials can provide meaningful information for making the antibiotic selection.[6–8,11] It is imperative that field trials be properly designed and conducted, and statistical analysis should always be done. An explanation of the background and class of cattle, management conditions, and details on the time-event relationships provide important details to the practitioner. Field trials evaluate antimicrobials under "real" conditions. Random microbiologic testing should be done to define the causative agent and antibiotic sensitivity or resistance. Many practitioners have criticized field trials for "not being representative" of cattle they care for, but field trial data are much more controlled and objective than are clinical impressions. Unfortunately, there is a paucity of well-controlled, published field trials to provide information to the practitioner and producer.

The last method used to select antimicrobial treatment for BRD is evaluation of clinical response. Detailed, accurate, current records should be kept and evaluated for response rate, relapse rate, case fatality rate, chronic rate, and cost of treatment. When comparing the feedlot data with field trial results, caution must be exercised to ensure that nomenclature and use of statistics are understood as their usage is not consistent.[12] Feedlot data should also be used to determine if goals established by management and the veterinarian are met. Using clinical response rates as a criterion for antibiotic selection may appear on the surface to be an oversimplified method; however, it determines whether or not the treatment response is in line with industry standards and answers the basic question, "Does it work?"

Combination antimicrobial therapy is commonly used to treat stocker and feeder cattle with BRD. Combination therapy is given primarily to broaden the antibacterial spectrum so that potential bacterial resistance can be overcome and potential mixed bacterial infections can be more effectively treated. Nevertheless, in many cases it is used because of a lack of confidence in single drug therapy. In vitro studies have shown that combinations of antibacterials can have synergistic or additive benefits against *Pasteurella haemolytica* when compared to treatment with a single antimicrobial.[13] However, in several field trials in commercial feedyards comparing combination antimicrobial therapy to a single antibiotic, results indicate similar response rates, relapse rates, and case fatality rates; moreover, treatment costs were markedly higher when combination therapy was used.[14–17]

Several other factors influence antibiotic selection. Whenever possible, products approved by the Food and Drug Adminis-tration (FDA) should be used. Drugs should only be used in an extralabel manner if approved products and routes have been shown to be ineffective. Products used should not cause undue pain or swelling or cause injection site scarring in edible tissue. To avoid violative drug residues in cattle being marketed, antimicrobials that have predictable withdrawal times compatible with current management and marketing systems should be selected. Cost of the treatment program is also an important consideration.

ANCILLARY THERAPY

A wide array of products are used as ancillary or supportive therapy for calves with BRD. Unfortunately, these products are used mostly on an empirical basis as there is very little scientific evidence to justify their administration. Antihistamines are commonly used, but histamines do not play a major role in fibrinous pneumonia or bronchopneumonia.[9]

Glucocorticoids and nonsteroidal antiinflammatory drugs are often advocated as ancillary treatment for BRD. These drugs counteract the effects of eicosanoids, mediators of the inflammatory response. Glucocorticoids have potent antiinflammatory properties but are also potent suppressors of the immune system. The use of glucocorticoids for treating BRD reduces the response to antibiotic therapy and increases the relapse rate.[18] Their routine use in calves with BRD is contraindicated.

Nonsteroidal antiinflammatory drugs have antiinflammatory effects and are not immunosuppressive. Acetylsalicylic acid and phenylbutazone have not been adequately studied to justify their use as ancillary therapy for BRD.[19,20] Flunixin meglumine combined with oxytetracycline has shown advantages over tetracycline used alone in the treatment of BRD. The combination treatment resulted in higher feed intakes, earlier and steeper reductions of rectal temperatures, and an enhanced ability to clear *Pasteurella* from the lower airways.[21] Larger scale field trials need to be done in North American feedlot systems to evaluate the use of flunixin meglumine in natural BRD outbreaks. The cost and lack of FDA approval limit current use of this drug in the United States.

Vitamin injections are often used as ancillary BRD therapy. Multiple B vitamin injections seem to be most commonly employed, but there appears to be no scientific confirmation of any real benefit associated with their administration. Vitamin C, or ascorbic acid, has been shown experimentally to reduce the immunosuppressive effects of dexamethasone in calves[22]; however, no controlled clinical trials have been published to demonstrate their benefit under field conditions.

A review of the literature offers little support for commonly used ancillary therapy products. Antibacterial therapy is the major therapeutic defense against BRD losses. Good animal husbandry, including sick pen management, is likely of more value than the empirical use of ancillary therapy.

DETERMINATION OF TREATMENT RESPONSE

It is highly recommended that the veterinarian provide written protocols for treatment of stocker and feeder cattle. The protocol should include recommendations on when to initiate therapy for BRD, the antimicrobial to use, treatment response criteria that signal either a positive or negative response, and the secondary antimicrobial regimen to use if the primary method fails. Treated calves must be individually identified, and treatment records must be maintained. Without treatment records, the success or failure of the treatment program cannot be determined. A residue avoidance program must be rigidly followed to preclude marketing of cattle with violative residues.

When calves are initially treated, baseline information (discussed below) should be recorded, which allows changes in the calves' condition to be evaluated. Two protocols for treatment of BRD are worthy of discussion here. The first protocol was described by Hjerpe and Routen[23] several years ago but remains a classic today:

■ As each animal is treated for the first time, a prenumbered tag is placed in the ear. This number is written on an individual cattle medication record card or entered into the computer along with the lot number, the date, the rectal temperature, the degree of sickness, and the medication used.

■ Under "degree of illness," the animal is assigned a number that designates degree of severity (ranging from 3 = moderately ill [moderately depressed; gaunt] to 1 = slightly ill to almost normal).

■ Twenty-four hours later, the rectal temperature and the "degree of illness" are again determined and recorded on the animal's card and the initial treatment is repeated.

■ Forty-eight hours after initial treatment, the rectal temperature and "degree of illness" are again determined and recorded. The 24 and 48 hour findings are then compared with the initial rectal temperature and "degree of illness" to determine if a favorable response has occurred. If the animal is definitely better, the original antimicrobial is readministered daily (as long as improvement continues) until fever, depression, weakness, heavy breathing, and inappetence are absent for two consecutive examinations. In most cases, absence of fever is defined as a rectal temperature of 103.0° F or less. The following criteria are used in judging response to treatment and in deciding whether or not to continue treatment with a given antimicrobial:

— If the initial rectal temperature was greater than 104.0° F, a reduction to 103.5° F or less within 48 hours is indicative of a favorable response.

— If the initial rectal temperature was between 103.0° and 104.0° F, progressive reduction toward 103.0° F is indicative of a favorable response. However, if the rectal temperature remains above 103.1° F on three consecutive days, with no tendency to decline toward 103.0° F, the treatment should be changed.

— If, during treatment with a given antimicrobial, the rectal temperature should fall to 103.0° F or less, the drug should be administered again on the following day, even though the rectal temperature may rebound. On the day following the rebound, the treatment should be changed unless there has been a reduction in the fever to 103.5° F or less.

— If the initial rectal temperature was less than 103.0° F, an improvement in the degree of illness rating is indicative of a favorable response.

— If evidence of a favorable response (as previously defined) is lacking after the mandatory number of treatments with a particular antimicrobial, the treatment should be changed.

— When treating cases in which (a) relapses have occurred two or more times or (b) response does not occur within the first 3 days after initiation of therapy, treatment should be continued until fever, depression, weakness, heavy breathing, and inappetence are absent on three to five (or more) consecutive examinations, depending on the general health and past history of the individual.

More recently, another method has been investigated that approached treatment management from a slightly different angle, as described below[14]:

■ Place eartag in the ear.
■ Assign a degree of illness score as previously described.
■ Take body temperature.
■ Treat with the drug of choice.
■ Repeat treatment, score the severity of illness, and take the rectal temperature on days 2 and 3.
■ On day 4, evaluate and look for improvement in severity score and body temperature. If the animal is considered well, discontinue treatment. If the animal's condition has not improved or has worsened, change to the second drug in the sequence. If the animal's condition has improved but it is not considered well, continue the initial treatment on days 4 and 5.
■ Day 6—If the animal is considered well, discontinue treatment. If it is not, consider changing the antimicrobial.

Results of studies[14] using this technique showed that only 72% to 75% of the treated calves were considered well after 3 days of treatment, whereas the response rates were at 96% or greater when the calves were treated for two more days with the same drug. These data suggest quite strongly that many stressed calves benefit from 5 days of treatment rather than the standard 3 days. This system has the potential to reduce the number of times antimicrobials need to be switched in treatment programs.

Either of these two systems can be adapted for use with single-injection, sustained-release antibiotics currently available. Currently, my personal treatment approach is to reevaluate treated calves at 48 hours following initial treatment. Calves that show improvement but that are not considered well are treated again at 48 hours with the same drug used initially. Therapy is changed at 48 hours if the calf's condition has not improved or has worsened. The withdrawal time is extended beyond FDA recommendations if a second injection of a sustained-release product is given. Controlled studies would be helpful to confirm or refute this method of therapeutic management.

There is disagreement among veterinarians and among researchers about the relative value of rectal temperatures and clinical evaluation for determining response to BRD therapy. Some have proposed that body temperature should drop below 103.5° F before cessation of treatment,[11,23] while many practitioners and feedlot consultants use visual evaluation as the primary basis for stopping treatment. Visual evaluation is more commonly used when long-acting antimicrobials are used. This takes advantage of the need for fewer trips through the chute and lower labor requirements, important considerations when hospital numbers are high.

The selection of the antimicrobial for treatment of relapses has also been debated. One approach is as follows: If a relapse occurs within 30 days after a previous illness, reinstitute the treatment to which the cattle previously responded; if more than 30 days have elapsed, start with the first drug outlined in the treatment sequence.[23] In many life-threatening cases of BRD, all antibacterials in the treatment sequence are quickly used with no satisfactory response, resulting in cases being classified as chronic. It is obvious that there is a point in the treatment process where administration of continued therapy to unresponsive patients is fruitless, but there is no consensus as to how much treatment is enough.

EVALUATION OF TREATMENT SUCCESS AND FAILURE

Treatment success can be measured by achieving industry standards and realistic feedlot goals for response rate, relapse rate, case fatality rate, and treatment costs. A response rate to the first drug of approximately 85% seems reasonable, although the rate may decline in the fall of the year, during inclement weather, and when higher numbers of high risk, stale cattle are received. Response rates to first therapy from controlled field trials have been reported to be about 85%[24–26] in cattle that are not extremely stale on arrival. In an Oklahoma study, a marked difference in response rate was seen between groups of calves that were received during the same time frame in the same backgrounding yard and treated with the same antimicrobial regimen. One group had an 86.1% response to first therapy and the other group had only a 54.9% response rate.[26] The latter group of calves were much lower priced and took considerably longer to assemble than the former group. There are variations in response rates between groups of cattle years and seasons of the year, as well as differences among feedlots.[2,11,24] While cattle owners and veterinarians have traditionally blamed antimicrobial resistance for this variation, other factors strongly influence response rates and case fatality rates.

Calves treated for BRD within 5 days of arrival have high relapse rates and high case fatality rates.[24,27] Likewise, cattle that die of BRD within 4 days of being pulled from the home pen are either pulled late or were received sick.[4,27] Late treatment is the single most important cause for respiratory disease treatment failure.[4] When more than 50% to 60% of a calf's lungs are consolidated, treatment is nearly always unsatisfactory.[5]

A review of the literature indicates that case fatality rates due to BRD are quite variable. Based on analysis of treatment records, I have established a goal of a 6% case fatality rate or less, but in the literature rates range from 1.4% to nearly 15%.[24,26] Several factors influence case fatality rates. As with response rates, cattle pulled late for treatment or sick on arrival are at greater risk of dying. Inadequate duration of therapy or improper drug dosage could result in a poor treatment response and higher case fatality rates.

Concurrent diseases, such as coccidiosis, salmonellosis, and viral diseases, can retard clinical response to therapy and increase death loss. In particular, bovine viral diarrhea virus (BVDV) infection is very immunosuppressive and impairs bacterial clearance from the lung, promotes dissemination of bacteria within the lung, and enhances the severity of disease caused by

Pasteurella haemolytica.[28,29] Direct correlation between BVDV infection and BRD has been reported.[30]

When a favorable treatment response is lacking, hospital pen management must also be evaluated. This area is often neglected; however, proper management is essential to a successful program. Shelter should be provided to protect the sick calf from extreme temperatures. The pen surface should be scraped frequently to ensure a favorable, comfortable environment. Overcrowding of feedlot hospitals is common, especially in the fall when large numbers of new cattle are received and morbidity rates are at their peak. Approximately 150 square feet per head should be provided. Transmission of enteric disease, especially salmonellosis, is not uncommon when pens are overcrowded or unsanitary.

Nutritional management of sick cattle is essential. Good quality grass hay should be available, and many nutritionists formulate a special, highly palatable ration for hospitalized cattle. A minimum of 12 inches of bunk space per head should be provided. Care must be taken to avoid overfeeding hospitalized cattle as the feed quickly becomes stale and further retards appetite. Water tanks should be cleaned at least daily. Calves that are no longer being treated should be moved to the home pen or to a convalescent pen to minimize crowding and to further reduce the spread of disease.

Personnel responsible for the hospital area must check hospitalized cattle at least twice daily for relapses. Ignoring or delaying treatment in cattle that have experienced relapses results in more chronic cases or higher death losses.

SUMMARY

Prevention of disease is the primary objective of a health management program. Some cases of BRD will still occur. To successfully manage cattle that experience BRD, a well-constructed treatment plan should be in place. This plan should detail disease surveillance, diagnostics, monitoring of treatment failures, and therapeutic regimens. The plan must be scientifically based, consider animal welfare and the economics of the treatment program, and include residue avoidance procedures. Good records, frequently analyzed, help determine if the health program is meeting predicted goals and industry standards. The treatment program cannot stand alone but must be integrated into the total management scheme.

Finally, the people who care for these animals must be properly trained, motivated, and assigned a reasonable workload. In the end, it is these individuals and their decisions that affect the outcome.

REFERENCES

1. Crenshaw GL: Comments on control and management of diseases in beef cattle. *JAVMA* 152:923, 1968.
2. Jensen R, Pierson RE, Braddy PM, et al: Diseases of yearling feedlot cattle in Colorado. *JAVMA* 169:497–499, 1976.
3. Martin SW, Bohac JG: The association between serological titers in infectious bovine rhinotracheitis, bovine virus diarrhea, parainfluenza-3 virus, respiratory syncytial virus and treatment for respiratory disease in Ontario feedlot calves. *Can J Vet Res* 50:351–358, 1986.
4. Janzen ED, Stockdale PHG, Acres SD, Babiuk LA: Therapeutic and prophylactic effects of some antibiotics on experimental pneumonic pasteurellosis. *Can Vet J* 25:78–81, 1984.
5. Hjerpe CA: The bovine respiratory disease complex, in Howard JL (ed): *Current Veterinary Therapy: Food Animal Practice*, ed 3. Philadelphia, WB Saunders, 1993, pp 653–664.
6. Martin SW, Meek AH, Curtis RA: Antimicrobial use in feedlot calves; its association with culture rates and antimicrobial susceptibility. *Can J Comp Med* 47:6–10, 1983.
7. Martin SW, Meek AH: The interpretation of antimicrobial susceptibility patterns. *Can J Comp Med* 45:199–202, 1981.
8. Prescott JF, Baggot JD: Antimicrobial susceptibility testing and antimicrobial drug dosage. *JAVMA* 187:363–368, 1985.
9. Clarke CR, Burrows GE, Ames TR: Therapy of bovine bacterial pneumonia. *Vet Clin North Am Food Anim Pract* 7:669–694, 1991.
10. Libal MC: Comparison of minimum inhibitory concentration and disk-diffusion antimicrobic sensitivity testing of bacterial pathogens isolated from food animals. *Am J Vet Res* 46:1200–1205, 1985.

11. Mechor GD, Jim GK, Janzen ED: Comparison of penicillin, oxytetracycline, and trimethoprim-sulfadoxine in the treatment of undifferentiated bovine respiratory disease. *Can Vet J* 29:438–443, 1988.

12. Kelly AP, Janzen ED: Morbidity and mortality rates—Handle with care. *Can Vet J* 30:170–172, 1989.

13. Burrows GE, Ewing P: In vitro assessment of the efficacy of erythromycin in combination with oxytetracycline or spectinomycin against *Pasteurella haemolytica. J Vet Diagn Invest* 1:299–304, 1989.

14. A comparative evaluation of Naxcel sterile powder for treatment of bovine respiratory disease under field conditions. Upjohn Veterinary Report No 2.

15. A comparison trial of Naxcel sterile powder to a combination of spectinomycin and erythromycin for treatment of bovine respiratory disease (BRD). Upjohn Veterinary Report No 3.

16. Therapy comparisons for bovine respiratory disease in Northwestern US feedlots. Upjohn Veterinary Report No 8.

17. Therapy comparisons for bovine respiratory disease in feedlots in the high plains. Upjohn Veterinary Report No 10.

18. Christie BM, Pierson RE, Braddy PM, et al: Efficacy of corticosteroids as supportive therapy for bronchial pneumonia in yearling feedlot cattle. *Bovine Pract* 12:115–117, 1977.

19. Apley MD: Ancillary therapy for bovine respiratory disease. Proceedings of the 26th Annual Conference of the American Association of Bovine Practitioners, 1993, pp 124–130.

20. Gingerich DA, Baggot JD, Yeary RA: Pharmacokinetics and dosage of aspirin in cattle. *JAVMA* 167:945–948, 1975.

21. Selman IE, Allan EM, Dalgleish RG, et al: The effects of flunixin meglumine and oxytetracycline therapy alone and in combination in calves with experimentally-induced pneumonic pasteurellosis. Proceedings of the 14th World Congress on Diseases of Cattle, Dublin, Ireland, 1986, pp 606–610.

22. Roth JA, Kaeberle ML: In vitro effect of ascorbic acid on neutrophil function in healthy and dexamethasone-treated cattle. *Am J Vet Res* 46:2434–2436, 1985.

23. Hjerpe CA, Routen TA: Practical and theoretical considerations concerning treatment of bacterial pneumonia in feedlot cattle, with special reference to antimicrobic therapy. Proceedings of the 9th Annual Conference of the American Association of Bovine Practitioners, 1976, pp 97–140.

24. Bateman KG, Martin SW, Shewen PE, Menzies PI: An evaluation of antimicrobial therapy for undifferentiated bovine respiratory disease. *Can Vet J* 31:689–696, 1990.

25. Smith RA, Gill DR, VanKoevering MT: Effects of tilmicosin or ceftiofur on health and performance of stressed stocker cattle. OSU Animal Science Research Report P-933, 1993, pp 308–311.

26. Smith RA, Gill DR, VanKoevering MT: A comparison of tilmicosin and ceftiofur for the treatment of bovine respiratory disease. *Bovine Pract* 28:35–37, 1994.

27. Deyhle CE Jr: Processing, handling, pen riding, pulling sick cattle and sampling procedures, in Albin RC, Thompson GB (eds): *Cattle Feeding: A Guide to Management.* Amarillo, TX, Trafton Printing, 1990, pp 169–177.

28. Potgieter LND: Immunosuppression in cattle as a result of bovine viral diarrhea virus infection. *Agri-Practice* 9(5):7–14, 1988.

29. Clarke CR, Short CR, Corstvet RE, Nobles D: Interaction between *Pasteurella haemolytica,* sulfadiazine/trimethoprim and bovine virus diarrhea. *Am J Vet Res* 50:1557–1565, 1989.

30. Reggiardo C: Role of BVD virus in shipping fever of feedlot cattle. Case studies and diagnostic consideration. *Am Assoc Vet Lab Diagn* 22:315–320, 1979.

Review of Bovine Respiratory Disease: Nutrition and Disease Interactions[a]

N. Andy Cole, PhD, Supervisory Research Animal Nutritionist
Conservation and Production Research Laboratory
Agricultural Research Division
U.S. Department of Agriculture
Bushland, Texas

Feeder calves encounter numerous physiologic and psychologic stressors (e.g., feed and water deprivation, weaning, inclement weather, antagonistic encounters, infectious agents, and transport) during movement from one production point to another. These stressors induce hormonal changes, anorexia, exhaustion, nutrient losses, altered nutrient metabolism, dehydration, behavioral changes, and immunosuppression. The adverse effects of many of these stressors seem to be additive. Affected calves present special nutritional, management, and health challenges to cattle producers and consultants.

Inadequate nutrition can accentuate the adverse effects of stress. Although proper nutrition generally cannot prevent stress or infection, it may have both direct and indirect beneficial effects on the animal. Proper nutrition can assist in preparing the animal for a period of stress, can decrease the adverse effects of stress, and can enhance recovery from stressful periods. Thus proper nutrition can help prevent the immunosuppression caused by stress.

INTERRELATIONSHIPS AMONG STRESS, NUTRITION, AND IMMUNITY

Basic Concepts

The immune system of mammals consists of three components:

- Mucosal barrier immunity
- Humoral immunity (antibodies)
- Cell-mediated immunity

Although often discussed separately, each component is intricately linked to the other two. Nutrition can affect many aspects of the immune system, among them (1) anatomic development of lymphoid tissues, (2) mucus production, (3) synthesis of immunologically active substances, (4) cellular proliferation, (5) cellular activation and movement, (6) intracellular killing, and (7) modulation and regulation of immune processes.[1]

In general, severe nutrient deficiencies impair at least one of the three components of the immune system (Table 1), but even subclinical deficiencies can impair immune response.[2] Much of the research concerning the interrelationship between nutrition and immunity is complicated by the fact that nutritional modification may have positive effects on one immune component while having negative effects on others. This suggests that modifications in nutrition that can be beneficial in protecting the animal from a specific virus at the same time may have adverse effects on the animal's ability to avoid a bacterial infection.

The "real world" value of much of the data concerning the effects of specific nutritional deficiencies and excesses on components of the immune system is often unclear. For example, are data collected on normal subjects applicable to those subjects when numerous stressors have had deleterious effects on their immune system? At what point is a depression in a specific immune

[a]The mention of trade or manufacturer names is made for information only and does not imply an endorsement, recommendation, or exclusion by USDA-Agricultural Research Service.

TABLE 1

Summary of the Effects of Nutritional Supplementation of Deficient Diets on Immune Response and Feeder Calf Health

Nutrient	CMI	Humoral	% BRD
		Immune Component	
Protein			
Chronic	D	NE, I	?
Acute	I, D	I, D	D
Protein-calorie	I	I	D
Vitamins			
A	—	I	NE
D	—	NE	NE
E	I	I	I, NE, D
C	I	I	
B_1	NE	I	NE, D
B_{12}	I	I	NE, D
Minerals			
Iron	I	—	—
Zinc	I	—	NE, D
Selenium	I	I	NE, D
Copper	I	I	—
Iodine (thyroxine)	I	NE, I	NE
Chromium	?	?	D?
Amino acids	I	I	—

CMI = cell-mediated immunity; % BRD = percentage of calves treated for bovine respiratory disease; I = increased; D = decreased; NE = no effect; ? = variable data; — = insufficient data. From Chandra RK: *Ann NY Acad Sci* 587:9–16, 1990 and References 6, 8, 21–22, 50, 52–55, 73–86, and 92–96.

component large enough to actually decrease the animals' ability to fend off a natural infection? Do short-term nutritional deficiencies have adverse effects on immunity?

Stress Effects on Nutrient Metabolism, Endocrine Response, Feed Intake Regulation, and Nutrient Requirements

Numerous metabolic changes occur in calves during marketing/transport (Table 2). Some stressors (e.g., infection) induce a hypermetabolic state in which nutrient balance is decreased, even if there is no decrease in nutrient intake.[3] Although many of these metabolic changes can be corrected in 1 or 2 days, others require as long as 14 days for complete correction. The nutritionist therefore has two principal objectives in feeding the stressed feeder calf: (1) decrease or prevent metabolic changes and (2) speed recovery without causing other deleterious effects.

Accomplishment of these objectives is complicated by low feed intakes during marketing and the first 1 to 2 weeks after arrival at the feedyard. These low feed intakes are caused by a combination of decreased ruminal function and metabolic adaptations that occur during stress.[4–7] Nonetheless, partial compensation for the stress-induced hypermetabolic state can be made by an increase in nutrient density of the diet.[8]

One of the most obvious metabolic changes that occurs during marketing/transport is weight loss (shrink). Even in short-haul (less than 6 hours) cattle, approximately 50% of weight loss involves gut contents and approximately 50% involves tissue loss.[9,10] In general, a 24 hour transport peri-

TABLE 2

Influence of Stress on Selected Metabolic Characteristics

Variable	Fasting	Transport	Infection
Nitrogen and phosphorus balance	D	D	D
Feed intake	D	D	D
Ruminal fermentation	D	D	D?
Serum insulin	D	?	I[a]
Serum growth hormone	NE[b]	?	?
Serum T_3 and T_4	D	D?	D
Plasma urea nitrogen	I	I?	D
Plasma glucose	I, D	I, D	I, D
Serum phosphorus	I?	D	D
Serum copper	NE	?	I
Serum zinc	I, D	?	D
Serum iron	D	D	D
RBC hemolysis	I?	I	?
Immune variables			
WBC count	D	I	I, D
Blastogenesis	?	D	?
Parasite shedding	?	I	?

I = increase; D = decrease; NE = no effect; ? = insufficient data or highly conflicting data; T_3 = triiodothyronine; T_4 = thyroxine.

[a]Accompanied by decreased glucose tolerance.

[b]Baseline concentrations are not affected, but response to feeding or glucose infusion is markedly altered.

od has the same metabolic effects as a 48 to 72 hour feed and water deprivation period.[10–12] The major stressors associated with transport seem to be loading and noise.[10–13] If ruminants are well fed before a fasting/transport period, there seem to be sufficient quantities of Ca, Mg, Na, Cu, Zn, and Fe in the gastrointestinal tract to prevent excessive losses of these nutrients from the tissues. However, tissues must be used as a source of some other nutrients (P, K, N, and water).[14]

PRACTICAL NUTRITION OF STOCKER/FEEDER CALVES

Feeding prior to the Stress of Marketing/Transport

Ruminants have a potentially large reserve of nutrients and water within the digestive tract. Increased performance and decreased morbidity and mortality can be realized if maximum use is made of this reserve.[15] Hence, the diet fed to calves before a stress period can be critical in determining their post-stress health and performance.

The diet of feeder calves at the farm of origin usually consists of grass and milk. Between the ages of 140 to 210 days, calves receive about 81% of their digestible energy intake from grass and about 19% from milk.[16] As a result, the diet calves receive at the farm/ranch can be highly variable, depending on the quality and quantity of grass available. Other factors such as plant toxins like the fescue endophyte *(Acremonium coenophialum)* may adversely affect nutrient[17] and immune[18,19] status of calves when they leave the farm of origin.

One method to ensure that calves are properly nourished upon leaving the farm is to wean them 4 weeks before sale and feed

TABLE 3
A 17 Trial Summary of the Effects of Preweaning and/or Preconditioning for 30 Days on Feeder Calves[a]

Parameter	Trials	Control	Preconditioned
On farm (last 30 days)			
Weight gain (lb)	17	43	48
Feed intake (lb)	12	0	363
Feed/added gain (lb/lb)	12	—	79.2
Transport shrink (%)	10	8.75	9.00
Feedyard performance			
Daily gain (lb)	13	2.34	2.32
Feed/gain (lb/lb)	7	7.17	7.48
Morbidity (%)	15	38.6	30.5
Mortality (%)	15	2.0	1.2

[a]See References 23 and 24 for data sources.

a balanced ration (preweaning). Practically, however, this procedure requires considerable extra time, labor, investment, risk, and skills by the cow-calf producer. Except when grass conditions are very poor, preweaning does not substantially benefit the cow herd.[20] Controlled research studies tend to indicate that, on average, calves preweaned and fed ad libitum for 30 days do not have sufficient improvements in either health or performance at the feedyard for the cattle feeder to pay a premium for the preweaning and feeding[21–26] (Table 3). On average, these calves gained 30 to 60 lb and consumed 200 to 500 lb of a 50% concentrate diet, whereas calves left with the cow and provided no supplemental feed gained 10 to 50 lb during the same period. At the feedyard, preweaned calves have about 20% less morbidity and death loss but 0 to 7% poorer feed conversions than calves that were not preweaned. Thus, on average, economic benefits realized from improved health were negated by poorer feed conversions. More recent empirical evidence suggests that preweaning calves 45 to 60 days before sale and feeding them so that they gain about 2 lb per day is more economical than a 30 day ad libitum preweaning program.[27] It is also likely that preweaning large-framed calves is more

economical than preweaning small-framed ones.

A second method of providing proper nutrition for calves at the farm that requires less investment and time than preweaning and feeding is creep feeding. Best returns seem to occur when calves are creep fed for about the last 60 days at the farm. Poorer economic returns occur when the creep feeding period is shorter or longer than 60 days.[28] Creep feeding of "large-framed" calves seems to be more economically profitable than creep feeding of "small-framed" calves.[29]

Several studies indicate that the best economic returns occur when calves are limit fed during the creep period[30–35] (Table 4). Providing each calf daily with 1 to 3 lb of a creep ration formulated to balance for grass conditions can yield a 0.2 to 0.5 lb per day increase in calf weight gain. Once calves learn to eat the creep ration, intakes can be limited via the use of salt.[31] Limited creep rations have ranged from a simple 90% cottonseed meal/10% salt mixture to very complex formulations.

Limited creep feeding of calves can be difficult to manage, and some producers object to the high salt concentrations often required in the creep ration to limit intakes. However, studies in Florida indicate that

TABLE 4
Influence of Limited Creep Feeding on Feeder Calves

Study and Parameter	Control	Creep	Preconditioned
Pate and Crockett[30]			
Sale weight (lb)	508	513	497
Daily gain (lb)	1.91	2.20	2.05
Morbidity (%)	26	2	10
Mortality (%)	2	0	0
Lusby[31]			
Preweaning ADG (lb)	1.16	1.42	
Creep feed/added gain (lb/lb)	—	5.5	
Transport shrink (lb)	11.7	19.8	
Feedlot ADG (lb)	2.09	2.29	
Treatments/calf	3.2	2.6	

ADG = average daily gain.

TABLE 5
Response of Florida Calves to Limited Creep Feeding of Cottonseed Meal or Molasses for 60 Days

Parameter	Control	Cottonseed Creep	Molasses Creep
Creep intake (lb/day)	—	0.44	0.77
Daily gain (lb)	1.46	1.68	1.87
Added gain (lb/day)	—	0.22	0.41
Feed/added gain (lb/lb)	—	2.00	1.88
Cost/added gain ($/lb)	—	0.26	0.09

Data from T. Weaver, U.S. Sugar Corp.

molasses-based, liquid creep feeds can be used very successfully[b] (Table 5). Compared to grain-based creep feeds, liquid creep feeds can be easier to manage, require less labor, do not require high salt concentrations to limit intake, and may be more easily adjusted to control intake.

Results of one study indicate that limited creep fed calves have about 20% to 25% less morbidity and death loss and 0 to 3% better feed conversions at the feedyard.[30] Thus, from a practical standpoint, limited creep feeding offers many advantages over a preweaning program under most circumstances.

[b]Weaver T: Personal communication.

Feeding during Marketing/Transport

Because of costs and logistics, most auction and order-buyer facilities provide calves with a diet of only low quality hay; properly formulated diets and supplements are usually not available. Compared to calves fed a low quality hay, calves fed a nutritionally balanced, 50% concentrate pretransport diet lose about 30% less weight, 25% less water, and 30% less protein during a 24 hour transport period.[10,11] In addition, calves fed a nutritionally balanced diet while in the auction or order-buyer facility have lower morbidity and better feedyard performance than calves fed low

TABLE 6
Effects of Order-Buyer Barn Diet[a] on Feedlot Performance[b]

Parameter	Hay	50% Concentrate Diet	Improvement
Daily gain (lb)	2.51	2.68	6.8%
Morbidity (%)	44.5	39.3	13.2%
Mortality (%)	6.15	2.99	51.4%
Feed/gain (lb/lb)	5.57	5.41	2.9%

[a]Diets were fed for 3 days before transport from Tennessee to Texas.
[b]Means of three studies (References 21 and 70 and Koers WC et al: *J Anim Sci* 41:408, 1975).

TABLE 7
Typical Dry Matter Intake (DMI) of Newly Arrived Feeder Calves

Days after Arrival	DMI (% of body weight)
1–7	0.5–1.5
8–14	1.5–2.5
15–28	2.5–3.5

Data from Hutcheson DP, Cole NA: *J Anim Sci* 62:555–560, 1986.

TABLE 8
Cumulative Percentages of Calves Eating during the First 7 Days after Arrival at the Feedyard

Day	Calves Eating (%) Healthy	Morbid
1	38.9	27.0
2	66.2	47.3
3	84.5	66.6
4	88.9	75.8
5	90.2	80.1
6	94.6	81.7
7	94.6	83.4

Data from Hutcheson DP, Cole NA: *J Anim Sci* 62:555–560, 1986.

quality hay (Table 6). However, some calves will not eat a 50% concentrate diet at the auction or order-buyer facility. Therefore, to assure that all calves receive nutrients at the auction or order-buyer barn, calves should be offered both a 50% concentrate diet and good quality hay at these facilities.

When offered both concentrate and hay, calves normally consume 0.5% to 1% of their body weight of the concentrate portion and 1% to 1.5% of their weight of the hay. As hay quality improves, hay intake increases relative to concentrate intake. If calves are accustomed to eating a concentrate diet (either because of previous creep feeding or preweaning), intakes of the concentrate portion will be greater. Most newly weaned calves eat only enough hay and/or concentrate to meet their maintenance energy requirements during the short stay in the auction or order-buyer barn.[21,22] Therefore the diet should be formulated so that requirements for other nutrients (protein, vitamins, and minerals) are met if intake is limited (about 1% of body weight).

When given a nutritionally balanced diet before an extended transport period, calves have an increased capacity to tolerate the stresses of transit, start on feed faster, and have fewer health problems at the feedyard. Economic analysis indicates that feeding a nutritionally balanced diet

TABLE 9
Dietary Nutrient Requirements for a 440 lb Medium-Framed Steer Calf Eating 1%, 2%, or 3% of Body Weight[a]

Parameter	Intake (% of Body Weight)		
	1%	2%	3%
Average intake (lb)	4.4	8.8	13.2
Expected daily gain (lb)[a]	−0.29	1.10	2.35
Required concentration			
Crude protein (%)	15.8	13.0	11.8
Calcium (%)	0.55	0.50	0.55
Phosphorus (%)	0.45	0.28	0.27
Magnesium (%)	0.25	0.12	0.10[b]
Potassium (%)	1.60	0.80	0.60[b]
Sodium (%)	0.20	0.10	0.08[b]
Copper (ppm)	20	10	8[b]
Manganese (ppm)	100	50	40[b]
Iron (ppm)	125	62	50[b]
Zinc (ppm)	75	38	30[b]

[a]For calculations, it is assumed that ration has an NEm value of 1.7 Mcal/kg (77 mcal/cwt) and an NEg value of 0.95 Mcal/kg (43 mcal/cwt).
[b]Recommended values for all beef cattle diets from National Research Council: *Nutrient Requirements of Beef Cattle*, ed 6, rev. Washington, DC, National Academy Press, 1984.

rather than low quality hay at the order-buyer barn can result in about a $20 return for each dollar invested.

Feeding after the Stress of Marketing/Transport

The diet fed during the first 2 to 4 weeks after arrival at the feedyard or stocker operation can significantly affect morbidity, mortality, performance, and cost of gain. There is probably no single best receiving program for the stressed calf. The optimum program for each group of calves depends on their background, the amount of stress encountered during marketing/transport, feed costs, and cattle costs.

One major problem in feeding the market/transport-stressed calf is low feed intakes (Tables 7 and 8). Feed intake of stressed calves is highly variable, and many calves do not obtain adequate intakes until the second or third week after arrival; this makes proper formulation of the diets difficult (Table 9).

Energy

Under most circumstances, energy is the first limiting nutrient in the diet of market/transport-stressed calves, primarily as a result of their low feed intakes. In general, as the energy concentration of the receiving diet increases, net energy intake increases, morbidity and mortality increase, performance improves, and the cost of gain decreases[36,37] (Table 10). The adverse health effects of feeding higher energy diets to stressed calves can be partially overcome by providing free choice, good quality hay along with the concentrate diet for the first 3 to 7 days after arrival[36,37] (Table 11). The number of days that hay is fed should be based on the health of the cattle. If alfalfa is used in the receiving program, it should be of average to good (not excellent) quality. If native hay or oat hay is fed, it should be of good to excellent quality.[36,37]

In operations with limited capacity to mix complete diets, calves can be fed good quality native hay, with each calf also

TABLE 10

Effect of Concentrate Level in Receiving Diet on Calf Health and Performance

Parameter	% Concentrate in Diet		
	25%	50%	75%
Morbidity (%)	47	49	57
Mortality (%)	4.57	2.35	4.65
Treatment days/calf	2.5	2.7	3.3
Daily gain (lb)	1.25	1.40	1.47
Feed/gain (lb/lb)	7.58	7.07	6.12
Relative cost/lb gain ($)	1.00	1.02	0.98

Data from References 36 and 37.

TABLE 11

Influence of Feeding No Hay, Free Choice Alfalfa Hay, or Free Choice Native Hay with a 75% Concentrate Receiving Diet on Feeder Calf Health and Performance

Parameter	No Hay	Alfalfa Hay	Native Hay
Morbidity (%)	41	37	30
Mortality (%)	0.9	0.0	0.9
Daily gain (lb)	1.02	1.12	0.90
Feed/gain (lb/lb)	7.99	8.04	9.64
Relative cost/lb gain ($)	1.00	0.84	0.89

Data from References 36 and 37.

receiving 2 lb of a pelleted, 40% protein supplement daily.[38] The major limitation of this system is poor early performance.[37]

Highly stressed calves seem to have a low tolerance to supplemental fat in the receiving diet. Adding 4% fat (tallow/vegetable oil blend) to the receiving diet of stressed calves improved animal performance[39] (Table 12); however, when morbid calves received 4% fat in the diet, mortality increased. This finding suggests that although fat can be used in the receiving diet, it should not be added to hospital pen diets.

Stressed calves prefer a dry diet over a diet high in corn silage but seem to adapt to a corn silage-based diet within 7 to 14 days.[40–45] The type of grain (corn versus wheat versus sorghum) in the receiving diet seems to have little effect on calf health or performance.[46–48]

Protein

The crude protein requirements of stressed calves do not appear to be appreciably greater than those of nonstressed calves.[49,50] Because of low feed intakes, however, the concentration of protein in the diet must be increased to meet the calves' requirements. In general, best results have been obtained in research studies when the receiving diet contained 13.5% to 14.5% crude protein.[49–55]

Stressed calves have a low tolerance for urea and other non–protein-nitrogen sources. Urea intakes should be limited to

TABLE 12
Effect of Added Fat in the Receiving Diet on Calf Health and Performance

Parameter	Added Fat (%) 0%	Added Fat (%) 4%
Morbidity (%)	60.2	57.8
Mortality (%)	8.4	12.0
Daily gain on day 56 (lb)	2.20	2.42
Feed/gain on day 56 (lb/lb)	6.09	5.61

Data from Reference 39.

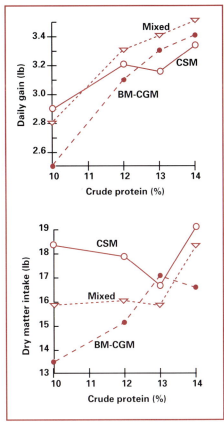

Figure 1. Effects of protein concentration and source on daily gain and dry matter intake of stressed feeder calves. CSM = cottonseed meal; BM-CGM = 50/50 blood meal/corn gluten meal; Mixed = mixture of 15% BM, 8% CGM, 33% hydrolyzed feather meal, 22% meat and bone meal, and 22% CSM.[54]

less than 30 g per head daily during the first 2 weeks after arrival.[56–58]

In general, feeding high "ruminal escape" (bypass) proteins to stressed calves has produced favorable results; however, improvements in health or performance are rarely sufficient to justify their high cost.[41,54,57,59–69] Calculations by Preston and Bartle[67] suggest that best results were obtained when about 60% of supplemental protein (i.e., 45% of total protein or 5.4% of diet dry matter) was composed of ruminal escape protein. The data of Brake and associates[54] suggest there may be an interaction between protein source and concentration in the receiving diet (Figure 1).

Minerals

As with protein, the mineral requirements of stressed calves do not seem to be appreciably increased compared to those of nonstressed calves. (One exception is potassium. The potassium requirement of stressed calves seems to be approximately 20% greater than nonstressed calves.[70]) However, the concentrations in the receiving diet must be increased to compensate for low feed intakes.

It is well documented that infection and stress affect trace mineral metabolism, especially Zn and Cu.[6,12,14,71–76] Nevertheless, studies on several trace mineral (Cu, Fe,

Zn, Se) requirements of stressed calves have been inconclusive. In addition, studies using organic/chelated forms of these minerals compared to inorganic forms have yielded variable or inconclusive results.[73–78] These highly variable results may be a result of interactions between trace mineral concentrations and sources.[77]

Numerous studies have been conducted to evaluate the effects of selenium supplementation on animal health, performance, and immune response.[79–83] As with

TABLE 13
Influence of Vitamin Supplementation on Feeder Calf Health and Performance

Vitamin(s) Given	Method of Administration	% Change with Supplementation		
		BRD	ADG	Gain/Feed
A and D	Injected	−3.0	+4.1	−1.1
A, D, and B_{12}	Injected	+3.0	+1.6	+2.4
A (11,000 IU/kg)	Fed	+28.0	−20.0	−9.0
Thiamine (1 g/head/day)	Fed	−17.0	+2.0	—
Niacin (250 ppm)	Fed	−4.0	+29.0	+45.0
B complex	Fed	−3.0	+4.2	+5.1
E (50 IU/head/day)	Fed	—	+5.3	—
E (100 IU/head/day)	Fed	—	+7.2	—
E (300 IU/head/day)	Fed	—	+14.0	—
E (400 IU/head/day)	Fed	−2.6	+5.2	+5.0
E (400 IU/head/day) + B complex	Fed	−0.5	+10.9	+10.9
E (800 IU/head/day)	Fed	−27.2	+38.4	+36.3
E (1600 IU/head/day)	Fed	−11.7	+22.2	+28.5
E (196 IU/kg)	Fed	—	+7.1	+0.3
E (340 IU/head)	Injected	−15.7	−10.8	−15.0
E (340 IU/head)	Injected	+14.3	+6.8	+10.0
E (1500 IU/head)	Injected	—	+14.3	—
E (1500 IU/head)	Injected	—	0.0	0.0
E (2000 IU/head)	Injected	+33.8	−1.2	−7.6
E (2500 IU/head)	Injected	+4.0	−1.9	—
E (3000 IU/head)	Injected	+12.6	−4.7	—

— = no data provided.
Data from References 21, 22, 54, 79, 81, 90–93, 96, and Hays VS et al: Oklahoma State University Animal Science Research Report MP-119, 1978, pp 198–201.

other trace minerals, experimental results have not been conclusive. Because Se use is regulated by federal agencies and there are concerns over its effect on the environment, Se supplementation should be monitored carefully and should be based on Se concentrations in basal ration ingredients.

Several recent studies have suggested that supplemental Cr may have beneficial effects on stressed calves.[84–86] As with Se, Cr is a potential environmental hazard; therefore supplementation should be monitored carefully.

Canadian workers demonstrated that providing electrolytes in the drinking water of slaughter bulls could increase hot carcass weight.[87,88] This suggests that provision of an electrolyte solution to market/transport-stressed calves might decrease tissue shrink. However, when lambs were subjected to stressors similar to those encountered by calves during marketing and transport, provision of an electrolyte solution did not affect the animal's response to stress.[89] Results at our location suggest that to obtain benefit from the provision of electrolyte solutions the concentration of electrolytes may need to be varied, depending on the level of stress encountered by the calf.[c]

[c]Cole NA: Unpublished data.

Vitamins

Studies testing the effects of injecting or feeding vitamins to stressed calves also have yielded variable results (Table 13). Some studies have shown dramatic improvements in health and performance,[90,91] whereas others have shown no effect[21,22,92] or even negative effects.

Feeding of B vitamins, especially niacin (100 to 200 ppm), has tended to decrease sickness and improve performance of stressed calves.[90,93] High intakes of vitamin E seem to stimulate the immune response if the vitamin is given before bacterial challenge but appear to have no effect when the vitamin is given after the challenge.[94,95] Most studies have noted improved performance and/or health of stressed calves fed supplemental vitamin E in the receiving diet. However, the performance and health responses of calves to injections of vitamin E have been more variable.[80,81,83,96] These variable results are probably due to the greater variability in the quality, composition, and recommended injection site (intramuscular versus subcutaneous) of the injectable vitamin E products that are available. Therefore producers and consultants should be wary and select injectable vitamin E products based on good research.

Other Nutritional Factors

A number of feed additives and supplements are currently available for use in stressed feeder calves. Both positive and negative data have been reported for most of these products. The use of feed additives in receiving diets must be based on need, efficacy, cost, and legality of combinations. Need and efficacy are usually determined by factors such as the source of the cattle, the amount of stress placed on the cattle, health of the cattle, weight and age of the cattle, season of the year, and the like.

The use of antibiotics in receiving diets has generally been associated with good results when morbidity and mortality were low.[97,98] When morbidity and mortality were high, use of antibiotics in the feed has been less promising, probably because calves did not consume enough of the ration containing the antibiotic. Variable response to prophylactic antibiotic treatment may be a result of the apparent increase in strains of *Pasteurella* resistant to many of the available antibiotics.[99,100]

Many stressed feeder calves excrete coccidia oocysts, and studies have indicated that the feeding of a coccidiostat upon arrival can be beneficial.[100–105] Best results with dietary coccidiostats have generally

TABLE 14
Recommended Nutrient Content of a Feedyard Receiving Diet for Market/Transport-Stressed Feeder Calves

Nutrient	Range
Dry matter (%)	82–90
NEm (mcal/cwt)	60–85[a]
NEg (mcal/cwt)	36–51[a]
Concentrate (%)	50–70[a]
Crude protein (%)	13.0–15.0
Urea (g/head/day)	<30
Calcium (%)	0.5–0.7
Phosphorus (%)	0.4–0.5
Potassium (%)	1.0–1.3
Sodium (%)	0.2–0.3
Magnesium (%)	0.2–0.3
Sulfur (%)	0.15–0.25
Manganese (ppm)	50–100
Copper (ppm)	10–20
Iron (ppm)	75–125
Zinc (ppm)	75–100
Selenium (ppm)	0.1–0.2
Cobalt (ppm)	0.1–0.2
Vitamin A (IU/lb)	1100–2000[b]
Vitamin E (IU/lb)	20–50[b]
Fat (%)	<6

[a]For calves weighing 400 lb or less use the greater value, for 500 lb calves use an intermediate value, and for 600 lb calves and yearlings use the lower value. Ration should be fed with free choice hay for the first 3 to 7 days.
[b]If pelleted, double the value to compensate for pelleting loss.

TABLE 15

Interaction between Vitamin E Injections and Vaccination with a *Pasteurella haemolytica* Toxoid

| Item | Nonvaccinated Calves | | Vaccinated Calves[a] | |
	Not Given Vitamin E	Given Vitamin E[b]	Not Given Vitamin E	Given Vitamin E[b]
Initial weight (lb)	382	382	378	378
Daily gain (lb)	1.66	1.65	1.75	1.74
Morbidity (%)	50	45	13	40
Treatment days/calf	2.0	2.5	2.5	1.9
Mortality (%)	6.7	3.4	0.0	3.3

Data from Reference 96.
[a]Calves vaccinated for *Pasteurella haemolytica* (IM) upon arrival at the feedyard.
[b]Calves injected IM with 2000 IU of vitamin E upon arrival.

been noted when morbidity and mortality were high.

The use of ionophores (monensin, lasalocid) upon arrival is complicated by the use of other additives such as antibiotics and coccidiostats. Addis and coworkers[106] recommended that monensin be limited to about 10 g per ton of receiving ration during the first 2 weeks. However, Prichard and Thompson[107] suggested that best results occurred when monensin was fed at 30 g per ton. Several studies have indicated that lasalocid in the receiving diet can have beneficial effects on performance.[101,108,109]

Most calves that enter feedyards carry a parasite burden, even if they are given an anthelmintic 30 days before shipment.[110] Because internal and external parasites can have marked effects on calf energy requirements,[111,112] calves should be treated for economically important helminth and arthropod parasites, even if the animals were "preconditioned."[113,114]

Some studies have shown beneficial effects of feeding (or dosing) *Lactobacillus,* yeast, and other microbial cultures upon arrival.[71,115–120] In general, the results have been variable and dose dependent. The use of these products in sick calves seems to be more promising than mass use in all incoming calves. The proportion of microorganisms that are destroyed by antibiotic treatment is not known.

A few studies have shown beneficial effects (on average, a 9% decrease in incidence of bovine respiratory disease and a 9% increase in daily gain) from daily feeding of 40 to 100 g of sodium bicarbonate per head upon arrival.[121–124]

Over the years, a number of commercial products have been reported to improve ruminal function and thereby improve feed intake, health, and performance. In general, the stress of administering these products is greater than the benefits achieved.[97,125] Our studies indicate that replacing the ruminal fluid of a stressed sheep with fluid from a nonstressed animal did not affect feed intake.[7] This is probably because metabolic, rather than ruminal, factors have the primary role in the control of feed intake in stressed calves.[4]

Suggested nutrient concentrations in a receiving diet for stressed feeder calves are presented in Table 14. As a general rule of thumb, receiving diets should be formulated so that the calf receives at least maintenance requirements for protein, vitamins, and minerals when feed consumption is 1% to 1.5% of body weight.

NUTRITIONAL AND MANAGEMENT INTERACTIONS

Interactions between common processing procedures (vaccination) and nutritional

TABLE 16
Interaction between Preshipment Management and Postshipment Diet Energy Concentration

Item	C-LE	PC-LE	C-HE	PC-HE
DM intake (lb)	14.7	15.2	12.3	14.5
DE intake (mcal)	14.7	15.0	16.7	19.6
Morbidity (%)	10.0	10.0	40.0	13.3

Data from Cole NA, Hutcheson DP, Ross JE, Thorne J: Unpublished data.
C = control calves left with their dam at the farm; PC = preconditioned calves, weaned and fed a 50% concentrate diet for 30 days before leaving the farm; LE = calves fed a low energy feedlot receiving diet; HE = calves fed a high energy receiving diet; DE = digestible energy.

regimens seem to occur[96] (Table 15). This suggests that some procedures that have normally been considered "good insurance" may in fact be detrimental to animal health and/or performance.

Management and nutritional factors that occur before the stress of marketing/transport can markedly influence which management and nutritional practices would be optimum after the animals' arrival at the feedyard. If calves have been consuming a high protein diet (e.g., lush grass) before transport, higher protein concentrations are required in the receiving diet.[49] Calves that have been accustomed to concentrate diets at the farm of origin (via preweaning or creep feeding) will eat more of a concentrate-based receiving diet than calves unaccustomed to concentrates but will eat about the same amount of high-roughage diets[d] (Table 16).

SUPPORTIVE NUTRITION

Many stressed and morbid calves refuse to eat any diet offered to them. Under these circumstances, as well as in cases involving severe diarrhea, it may become appropriate or necessary to provide supportive nutrition along with pharmaceutical treatment to keep the calf alive. In the morbid calf, simply decreasing body temperature may be adequate to stimulate the calf to eat. The use of certain microbial cul-

[d]Cole NA, Hutcheson DP, Ross JE, Thorne J: Unpublished data.

ture products containing *Lactobacillus acidophilus,* fungi, or yeast cultures may stimulate feed consumption in some animals. When these methods do not succeed, more strenuous measures such as intravenous, oral, intraruminal, or intraperitoneal infusions may be warranted.

Many oral and parenteral electrolyte and nutrient solutions are currently available. The advantages, disadvantages, and proper use of these solutions have been extensively reviewed elsewhere.[126]

CONCLUSIONS

Although general recommendations can be made concerning the preshipment and postshipment nutrition and management of stressed feeder calves, research data and practical experience indicate that no one program can be devised that is best for every load of calves. Hence the practitioner, consultant, and cattle feeder must be prepared to adjust management to fit each load of calves.

REFERENCES

1. Sherman AR: Influence of iron on immunity and disease resistance. *Ann NY Acad Sci* 587:140–147, 1990.
2. Rivlin RS: The clinical significance of micronutrients in relation to immune functions. *Ann NY Acad Sci* 587:55–59, 1990.
3. Cole NA, Delaney DD, Cummins JM, Hutcheson DP: Influence of experimental viral challenge on the nitrogen metabolism of calves. *Am J Vet Res* 47:1160–1165, 1986.
4. Cole NA, Purdy CW, Hallford DM: Influence

of fasting and postfast diet energy level on feed intake, feeding pattern, and blood variables of lambs. *J Anim Sci* 66:798–805, 1988.

5. Cole NA, Hallford DM, Gallavan R: Influence of a glucose load in fed or unfed lambs on blood metabolites and hormone patterns. *J Anim Sci* 71:765–773, 1993.

6. Cole NA, Gallavan RH, Rodriguez SL, Purdy CW: Influence of triiodothyronine injections on calf immune response to an infectious bovine rhinotracheitis virus challenge and nitrogen balance in lambs. *J Anim Sci* 72:1263–1273, 1994.

7. Cole NA: Effects of animal-to-animal exchange of ruminal contents on the feed intake and ruminal characteristics of fed and fasted lambs. *J Anim Sci* 69:1795–1803, 1991.

8. Boyles OW, Cobb CS, Cole NA, et al: Influence of protein status on the severity of the hypermetabolic response of calves with infectious bovine rhinotracheitis virus. *J Anim Sci* 67(Suppl 1):545, 1989 (abstract).

9. Self HL, Gay N: Shrink during shipment of feeder cattle. *J Anim Sci* 35:489–494, 1972.

10. Phillips WA, Cole NA, Hutcheson DP: The effect of diet on the amount and source of weight lost during transit or fasting. *Nutr Rep Int* 32:765–776, 1985.

11. Cole NA, Phillips WA, Hutcheson DP: The effect of prefast diet and transport on nitrogen metabolism of calves. *J Anim Sci* 62:1719–1731, 1986.

12. Cole NA, Camp TH, Rowe LD, et al: Effect of transport on feeder calves. *Am J Vet Res* 49:178–183, 1988.

13. Agnes F, Sartorelli P, Abdi BH, Locatelli A: Effect of transport loading or noise on blood biochemical variables in calves. *Am J Vet Res* 51:1679–1683, 1990.

14. Cole NA: Influence of feed and water deprivation on weight and composition of internal organs of lambs. *J Anim Sci* 72(Suppl 1):340, 1994 (abstract).

15. Cole NA, Hutcheson DP: Influence of prefast feed intake on recovery from feed and water deprivation by beef steers. *J Anim Sci* 60:772–779, 1985.

16. Bailey CB, Lawson JE: Estimated water and forage intakes in nursing range calves. *Can J Anim Sci* 61:415–421, 1981.

17. Stoszek MJ, Mika PG, Oldfield JE, Weswig PH: Influence of copper supplementation on blood and liver copper in cattle fed tall fescue or quackgrass. *J Anim Sci* 62:263–271, 1986.

18. Dew RK, Boissonneault GA, Gay N, Boling JA: Immune responses in Sprague-Dawley rats and mice fed endophyte infected tall fescue seed. *J Anim Sci* 66(Suppl 1):372, 1988 (abstract).

19. Purdy CW, Cole NA, Stuedemann JW: The effects of fescue toxicosis on classical complement in yearling feedlot cattle. *J Vet Diag Invest* 1:88, 1989 (abstract).

20. Basarab JA, Novak FS, Karren BP: Effects of early weaning on calf gain and cow performance and influence of breed, age of dam and sex of calf. *Can J Anim Sci* 66:349–358, 1986.

21. Cole NA, McLaren JB, Irwin MR: Influence of pretransit feeding regimen and posttransit B-vitamin supplementation on stressed feeder calves. *J Anim Sci* 49:310–319, 1979.

22. Cole NA, McLaren JB, Hutcheson DP: Influence of preweaning and B-vitamin supplementation of the feedlot receiving diet on calves subjected to marketing and transit stress. *J Anim Sci* 54:911–918, 1982.

23. Cole NA: Preconditioning calves for the feedlot. *Vet Clin North Am Food Anim Pract* 1:401–412, 1985.

24. Cole NA: Receiving nutrition and management for feedlots. *Proc XXV AABP* 2:309–315, 1992.

25. Ritchie H, Rust S: Does it pay to buy preconditioned feeder cattle? *Feedstuffs*, p 22, Apr 13, 1987.

26. Prichard RH, Mendez JK: Effects of preconditioning on pre- and post-shipment performance of feeder calves. *J Anim Sci* 68:28–34, 1990.

27. McNeill JW: 1992–93 Texas A&M Ranch-to-Rail Summary Report. Texas Agriculture Extension Service, College Station, TX, 1994.

28. Tarr SL, Faulkner DB, Buskirk DD, et al: The value of creep feeding during the last 84, 56, or 28 days prior to weaning on growth and performance of nursing calves grazing endophyte-infected tall fescue. *J Anim Sci* 72:1084–1094, 1994.

29. Anderson DC, O'Mary CC, Martin EL: Birth, preweaning and postweaning traits of Angus, Holstein, Simmental and Chianina sired calves. *J Anim Sci* 46:362–369, 1978.

30. Pate FM, Crockett JR: Feeding calves at weaning. Florida Beef Cattle Short Course, May 1974.

31. Lusby KS: Limit fed creep feeds for nursing calves. *Bovine Proc* 21:92–95, 1989.

32. Brazle FK, Kuhl GL, Binns CN, et al: The influence of limited-creep feeding on pre- and post-weaning performance of spring-born calves. *J Anim Sci* 69(Suppl 1):76, 1991 (abstract).

33. Cremin JD, Faulkner DB, Parrett DF, et al: Growth and feed efficiency of calves with restricted and unrestricted intake of creep feed. University of Illinois 1988–89 Beef Cattle Research Report, 1989, pp 21–26.

34. Cremin JD, Faulkner DB, Merchen NR: Effect of level and protein concentration of

creep feed on intake, digestibility and ruminal parameters of nursing calves. University of Illinois 1989–90 Beef Cattle Research Report, pp 35–41, 1990.

35. Hummel DF, Faulkner DB, Parrett DF, Buskirk DD: The effects of corn vs soy hulls limited vs ad libitum intake as a creep supplement on calf performance, subsequent performance during growing and finishing and carcass characteristics. University of Illinois 1990–91 Beef Cattle Research Report, pp 8–12, 1991.

36. Lofgreen GP: Nutrition and management of stressed beef calves. *Vet Clin North Am Large Anim Pract* 5(1):87–101, 1983.

37. Lofgreen GP: Nutrition and management of stressed beef calves: An update. *Vet Clin North Am Food Anim Pract* 4(3):509–528, 1988.

38. Smith RA, Hays VS, Gill DR: Management of stockers. *Agri-Practice* 9:8–14, 1988.

39. Cole NA, Hutcheson DP: Influence of receiving diet fat level on the health and performance of feeder calves. *Nutr Rept Int* 36:965–972, 1987.

40. Preston RL, Smith CK: Feedlot response of new feeder calves following a creep feeding period on the same or different protein source as that fed immediately after shipment. Ohio Agricultural Research and Development Center Research Summary 68, 1973, pp 33–35, 1973.

41. Preston RL, Smith CK: Role of protein level, protected soybean protein and roughage on the performance of new feeder calves. Ohio Agricultural Research and Development Center Research Summary 77, 1974, pp 47–50.

42. Preston RL, Kunkle WE: Role of roughage sources in the receiving ration of yearling feeder steers. Ohio Agricultural Research and Development Center Research Summary 77, 1974, pp 51–54.

43. Koers WC, Parrott JC, Sherrod LB, et al: Receiving and sick pen rations for stressed calves. Texas Tech University Research Report 25, 1975, pp 73–76.

44. Davis GV, Caley HK: Performance of stressed calves as influenced by management and ration. Kansas State University Roundup Report Bulletin 273, 1976, pp 17–21.

45. Davis GV, Caley HK: Influence of management and rations on the performance of stressed calves. Kansas State University Cattle Feeders Day Report of Progress 288, 1977, pp 16–20.

46. Brethour JR, Duitsman WW: Effect of zinc on dehorning stress. Kansas State University Roundup Report Bulletin 556, 1972, pp 39–42.

47. Addis D, Lofgreen GP, Clark JG, et al: Barley vs milo in receiving rations. California Cattle

Feeders Day Report, 1975, pp 53–58.

48. Addis D, Lofgreen GP, Clark JG, et al: Barley vs wheat in receiving rations for new cattle. California Cattle Feeders Day Report, 1978, pp 54–60.

49. Cole NA, Hutcheson DP: Influence of protein concentration in prefast and postfast diets on feed intake of steers and nitrogen and phosphorus metabolism of lambs. *J Anim Sci* 66:1764–1773, 1988.

50. Cole NA, Hutcheson DP: Influence of dietary protein concentrations on performance and nitrogen repletion in stressed calves. *J Anim Sci* 68:3488–3495, 1990.

51. Embry LB: Feeding and management of new feedlot cattle. South Dakota State University Cattle Feeders Day Report, 1977, pp 47–52.

52. Bartle SJ, Karr KJ, Ross JG, Preston RL: Supplemental protein sources and dietary crude protein level for receiving feedlot cattle. Texas Tech University Animal Science Research Report T-5-251, 1988, pp 61–62.

53. Eck TP, Bartle SJ, Preston RL, et al: Protein source and level for incoming feedlot cattle. *J Anim Sci* 66:1871–1876, 1988.

54. Brake AC, Preston RL, Bartle SJ: The role of protein level, source of ruminal escape protein and vitamin E on performance and blood parameters in newly received feeder cattle. Texas Tech University Animal Science Research Report T-5-317, 1992, pp 149–154.

55. Galyean ML, Gunter SA, Malcolm-Callis KJ, Garcia DR: Effects of crude protein concentration in the receiving diet on performance and health of newly received beef calves. New Mexico State University Clayton Research Center Progress Report 88, 1993.

56. Gates RN, Embry LB: Soybean meal or urea during feedlot adaptation and growing of calves. South Dakota State University Cattle Feeders Day, AS Series 7525, 1975, pp 27–33.

57. Preston RL, Byers FM, Moffitt PE, Parker CE: Soybean meal and urea as sources of supplemental protein for newly received feeder calves. Ohio Beef Day and Cattlemen's Roundup Report 8-75-5.5M:6–10, 1975.

58. Cole NA, Hutcheson DP, McLaren JB, Phillips WA: Influence of pretransit zeranol implant and receiving diet protein and urea levels on performance of yearling steers. *J Anim Sci* 58:527–533, 1984.

59. Grigsby ME: Protein supplementation for stressed calves. New Mexico State University Clayton Research Center Progress Report 25, 1981.

60. Phillips WA: Corn gluten meal plus urea for receiving steer and heifer calves. Oklahoma State University Animal Science Research Report MP-112, 1982, pp 77–80.

61. Phillips WA: The effect of protein source on

the poststress performance of steer and heifer calves. *Nutr Rept Int* 30:853–858, 1984.

62. Malcolm KJ, Duff GC, Galyean ML, Garcia DR: Effects of supplemental protein sources on performance of newly received calves. New Mexico State University Clayton Research Center Progress Report 71, 1991.

63. Zinn RA: Protein nutrition of lightweight stressed calves. *Desert Feedlot News,* July 1982.

64. Gunter SA, Galyean ML, Malcolm-Callis LJ, Garcia DR: Effects of origin of cattle and supplemental protein source on the performance of newly received feeder cattle. New Mexico State University Clayton Research Center Progress Report 85, 1993.

65. Zinn RA, Owens FN: Ruminal escape protein for lightweight feedlot calves. *J Anim Sci* 71:1677–1687, 1993.

66. Fluharty FL, Loerch SC, Smith FE: Effects of energy density and protein source on diet digestibility and performance of calves after arrival at the feedlot. *J Anim Sci* 72:1616–1622, 1994.

67. Preston RL, Bartle SJ: Quantification of rumen escape protein and amino acid needs for new feedlot cattle. Texas Tech University Agriculture Sciences Technical Report T-5-283, 1990, pp 17–19.

68. VanKoevering MT, Gill DR, Owens FN, et al: The effects of escape protein on health and performance of shipping stressed calves. Oklahoma State University Animal Science Research Report MP-134, 1991, pp 156–162.

69. VanKoevering MT, Gill DR, Owens FN, Ball RL: The effects of types and quality of protein on health and performance of shipping-stressed calves. Oklahoma State University Animal Science Research Report MP-136, 1992, pp 326–332.

70. Hutcheson DP, Cole NA, McLaren JB: Effects of pretransit diet and post-transit potassium levels for feeder calves. *J Anim Sci* 58:700–706, 1984.

71. Cole NA, Purdy CW, Hutcheson DP: Influence of yeast culture on feeder calves and lambs. *J Anim Sci* 70:1682–1690, 1992.

72. Orr CL, Hutcheson DP, Grainger RB, et al: Serum copper, zinc, calcium, and phosphorus concentrations of calves stressed by bovine respiratory disease and infectious bovine rhinotracheitis. *J Anim Sci* 68:2893–2900, 1990.

73. Chirase NK, Hutcheson DP, Thompson GB: Feed intake, rectal temperature, and serum mineral concentrations of feedlot cattle fed zinc oxide or zinc methionine and challenged with infectious bovine rhinotracheitis virus. *J Anim Sci* 69:4137–4145, 1991.

74. Chirase NK, Hutcheson DP, Thompson GB, Spears JW: Recovery rate and plasma zinc

and copper concentrations of steer calves fed organic and inorganic zinc and manganese sources with or without injectable copper and challenged with infectious bovine rhinotracheitis virus. *J Anim Sci* 72:212–219, 1994.

75. Nockels CF, Oebonis J, Torrent J: Stress induction affects copper and zinc balance in calves fed organic and inorganic copper and zinc sources. *J Anim Sci* 71:2539–2545, 1993.

76. Stabel JR, Spears JW, Brown TT: Effect of copper deficiency on tissue, blood characteristics, and immune function of calves challenged with infectious bovine rhinotracheitis virus and *Pasteurella haemolytica. J Anim Sci* 71:1247–1255, 1993.

77. Malcolm-Callis KJ, Galyean ML, Gunter SA, Garcia DR: Effects of different zinc sources and levels, with or without copper lysine, on performance of newly weaned calves. New Mexico State University Clayton Research Center Progress Report 83, 1993.

78. Brazle FK, Stokka G: The effect of Fourplex on gain and health of newly-arrived calves. Kansas State University Cattleman's Day Report of Progress 704, 1994, pp 46–47.

79. Hutcheson DP, Cole NA: Vitamin E and selenium for yearling feedlot cattle. *Fed Proc* 44:549, 1985 (abstract).

80. Reffett JK, Spears JW, Brown TT: Effect of dietary selenium and vitamin E on the primary and secondary immune response in lambs challenged with parainfluenza-3 virus. *J Anim Sci* 66:1520–1528, 1988.

81. Droke EA, Loerch SC: Effects of parenteral selenium and vitamin E on performance, health and humoral immune response of steers new to the feedlot environment. *J Anim Sci* 67:1350–1359, 1989.

82. Stabel JR, Spears JW, Brown TT, Brake J: Selenium effects on glutathione peroxidase and the immune response of stressed calves challenged with *Pasteurella haemolytica. J Anim Sci* 67:557–564, 1989.

83. Pollock JM, McNair J, Kennedy S, et al: Effects of dietary vitamin E and selenium on in vitro cellular immune responses in cattle. *Res Vet Sci* 56:100–107, 1994.

84. Chang X, Mowat DN: Supplemental chromium for stressed and growing feeder calves. *J Anim Sci* 70:559–565, 1992.

85. Moonsie-Shageer S, Mowat DN: Effect of level of supplemental chromium on performance, serum constituents, and immune status of stressed feeder calves. *J Anim Sci* 71:232–238, 1993.

86. Lindell SA, Brandt RT, Minton JE, et al: Supplemental chromium and revaccination effects on performance and health of newly weaned calves. Kansas State University Cattlemen's Day Report of Progress 704, 1994, pp 31–34.

87. Schaefer AL, Jones SDM, Tong AKW, Young BA: Effects of transport and electrolyte supplementation on ion concentrations, carcass yield and quality in bulls. *Can J Anim Sci* 70:107–119, 1990.

88. Schaefer AL, Jones SDM, Tong AKW, et al: Effects of post-transport electrolyte supplementation on tissue electrolytes, hematology, urine osmolality and weight loss in beef bulls. *Livestock Prod Sci* 30:333–341, 1992.

89. Apple JK, Minton JE, Parsons KM, Unruh JA: Influence of repeated restraint and isolation stress and electrolyte administration on pituitary-adrenal secretions, electrolytes, and other blood constituents of sheep. *J Anim Sci* 71:71–77, 1993.

90. Overfield JR, Hixon DL, Hatfield EE: Effect of nutritional treatment of "stressed" feeder calves. University of Illinois Cattle Feeders Day AS-6721, 1976, pp 28–33.

91. Lee RW: Effect of vitamin supplementation of receiving diets on the performance of stressed beef calves. Kansas State University Cattle Feeders Day Report of Progress 474, 1986, pp 14–17.

92. Zinn RA, Alvarez E: Influence of vitamin A and vitamin E supplementation on health and performance of crossbred calves during a 56-d receiving period. *J Anim Sci* 70(Suppl 1):313, 1992.

93. Byers FM: Niacin for ruminants. *Feed Management* 22:25, July 1980.

94. Ellis RP, Vorhies VN: Effect of supplemental dietary vitamin E on the serologic response of swine to an *Escherichia coli* bacteria. *JAVMA* 168:231–236, 1976.

95. Lewis KJ, Nockels CF, Barber TL, Walton TE: Vitamin E enhancement of the immune response in horses. Colorado State University Research Highlights General Series 960, 1976, pp 22–27.

96. Galyean ML, Duff GC, Malcolm KJ, Garcia OR: Effects of *Pasteurella haemolytica* vaccine and injectable vitamin E on the performance and health of newly received calves. New Mexico State University Clayton Research Center Progress Report 70, 1991.

97. Brethour JR, Duitsman WW: Management of newly arrived calves: AS-700, pen size, rumen fluid inoculation. Kansas State University Roundup Report Bulletin 545, 1971, pp 34–38.

98. Byers FM, Smith CK: Antibiotics and protein supplements in receiving rations for feeder calves. Ohio Agricultural Research and Development Center Research Summary 1976, pp 20–24.

99. Post KW, Cole NA, Raleigh RH: In vitro antimicrobial susceptibility of *Pasteurella haemolytica* and *Pasteurella multocida* recovered from cattle with bovine respiratory disease complex. *J Vet Diag* 3:124–126, 1991.

100. Chengappa MM, Rogers OP, Vorhies MW: Antimicrobial resistance among important bovine pathogens isolated at the KSU Veterinary Diagnostic Laboratory over two and a half years. Kansas State University Cattlemen's Day Report of Progress 678, 1993, pp 139–140.

101. Hicks RB, Smith RA, Gill DR, et al: The effect of mass-medication, lasalocid or decoquinate, and medical treatment on the gains and health of newly-arrived stocker and feeder cattle. Oklahoma State University Animal Science Research Report MP-117, 1985, pp 221–228.

102. Hutcheson DP, Cummins JM: The use of decoquinate in the receiving diets of stressed feeder calves. *Proc West Sect Am Soc Anim Sci* 33:181–185, 1982.

103. Lusby KS, Oltjen JE, Barnes KS, Stevens VL: Three study summary of Deccox in receiving-growing diets for newly arrived stocker cattle. *J Anim Sci* 61(Suppl 1):423–424, 1985 (abstract).

104. Brazle F: Effects of decoquinate on gain and health of newly-arrived stocker cattle. Kansas State University Cattlemen's Day Report of Progress 494, 1986, pp 69–72.

105. Smith SC, Lusby KS, Evicks TL, et al: The effect of Deccox on weight gain of newly weaned beef calves. Oklahoma State University Animal Science Research Report MP-127, 1989, pp 51–54.

106. Addis D, Lofgreen GP, Clark JG, et al: Rumensin in receiving rations for new cattle. California Cattle Feeders Day Report, 1987, pp 64–67.

107. Prichard RH, Thompson JU: Optimum monensin levels in feeder calf receiving diets. South Dakota State University Feeders Day Report, 1993, pp 62–68.

108. Davis GV: Effects of Aureomycin and Bovatec on the performance of feedlot calves. Kansas State University Cattle Feeders Day Report of Progress 416, 1982, pp 33–37.

109. Gill DR, Richey EJ, Owens FN, Lusby KS: Effect of lasalocid on weight gains of stocker steers. Oklahoma State University Animal Science Research Report MP-112, 1982, pp 85–86.

110. Szanto J, Mohan RN, Levine NO: Prevalence of coccidia and gastrointestinal nematodes in beef cattle in Illinois and their relation to shipping fever. *JAVMA* 144:741–746, 1964.

111. Jordan H, Cole NA, McCroskey JE: The influence of *Ostertagia ostertagia* and *Cooperia* infections on the energetic efficiency of beef steers fed a high concentrate ration. *Am J Vet Res* 38:1157–1160, 1977.

112. Cole NA, Guillot FG: Influence of *Psoroptes ovis* on the energy metabolism of heifer

calves. *Vet Parasitol* 23:285–292, 1987.

113. Davis GV: Parasitism in feedlot cattle. Proceedings of the 11th Annual Convention of the American Association of Bovine Practitioners, 1987, pp 134–137.

114. Brazle F: The effect of levamisole on the gain and health of stressed calves. *J Anim Sci* 69(Suppl 1):77, 1991 (abstract).

115. Hicks RB, Gill OR, Smith HA, Ball RL: The effect of microbial culture on health and performance of newly-arrived stocker cattle. Oklahoma State University Animal Science Research Report MP-118, 1986, pp 256–259.

116. Brethour JR: Probios for cattle. Kansas State University Roundup Report of Progress 399, 1981, pp 15–18.

117. Crawford JS, Carver L, Berger J, Dana G: Effect of feeding a living nonfreeze-dried *Lactobacillus acidophilus* culture on performance of incoming feedlot steers. *Proc West Sect Am Soc Anim Sci* 31:210–212, 1980.

118. Hutcheson DP, Cole NA, Keaton W, et al: The use of a living, nonfreeze-dried *Lactobacillus acidophilus* culture for receiving feedlot calves. *Proc West Sect Amer Soc Anim Sci* 31:213–215, 1980.

119. Gill OR, Smith HA, Ball RL: The effect of probiotic feeding on health and performance of newly arrived stocker cattle. Oklahoma State University Animal Science Research Report MP-119, 1987, pp 202–204.

120. Phillips WA, VonTungeln DL: The effect of yeast culture on the poststress performance of feeder calves. *Nutr Rept Int* 32:287–294, 1985.

121. Brethour JR, Duitsman WW: Sodium bicarbonate and/or thiamine in postweaning stress rations. Kansas State University Roundup Report of Progress 266, 1976, pp 35–40.

122. Brethour JR, Duitsman WW: Wheat or dehydrated alfalfa in starting rations. Kansas State University Roundup Report Bulletin 556, 1972, pp 38–42.

123. Brethour JR, Duitsman WW: Ascorbic acid, sodium bicarbonate and thiamine in postweaning stress rations. Kansas State University Beef Cattle Feeding Investigations Bulletin 569, 1973, pp 40–43.

124. Orr CL, Billingsley RD, Damron SW, et al: Effect of sodium bicarbonate on the performance of market and transportation stressed calves. *J Anim Sci* 49(Suppl 1):56, 1979 (abstract).

125. Koers WC, Parrott JC, Sherrod LB, et al: Force feeding and rumen status of heavily stressed calves. Texas Tech University Research Report 24, 1974, pp 80–82.

126. Roussel AJ: Fluid therapy, transfusion and shock therapy, in Howard JL (ed): *Current Veterinary Therapy 3: Food Animal Practice.* Philadelphia, WB Saunders, 1993, pp 2–8.

Feedlot Health and Management

Kelly F. Lechtenberg, DVM, PhD, President
Midwest Veterinary Services, Inc.
Oakland, Nebraska

Gerald L. Stokka, DVM, MS, Assistant Professor
Department of Animal Sciences
Kansas State University
Manhattan, Kansas

The principal goals of a feedlot health program are (1) to reduce losses due to disease, (2) to minimize disease outbreaks, (3) to enhance performance, and (4) to provide professional assistance in health management.[1] These goals can only be achieved if the capability exists to measure the results of decisions that are made with regard to the health program. The recording of various health data in a record system is the initial step in this process.

A *record system* is a set of facts written down or recorded and arranged in a regular, logical form. These types of systems have been given a variety of names, such as management decision systems and decision support systems. Record systems for livestock production operations provide an important recourse for management for analysis and subsequent intervention decisions.[2,3] Analysis of information collected and collated in a record system is at the very core of any successful health management or preventive health program.

Record systems may be computerized and/or manually kept. For any type of system the information should be relatively easy to collect, the system should be easy to use, and the data should provide meaningful information. Many automated systems have been developed that provide page after page of facts and information. Unless the information can be used to assist in management decisions, however, it has very little production value.

Handwritten record systems can be used in almost any type of production system. Most systems may need to be custom designed for a particular operation. One system that works well in beef cattle confinement production systems utilizes pen treatment cards (Figure 1). This system allows up to 24 head to be entered on a single card. The multiple animal card eliminates the voluminous amount of paper that can accumulate with single animal card systems.

Regardless of the type of system used, the information collected should provide three fundamental pieces of information, namely (1) identification of the individual animal as well as its pen or lot, (2) the reason that the animal was pulled from the pen, and (3) the treatment that was administered. Additional information that should be collected includes the number of cattle in the pen, the arrival date, the inweight of the cattle, and the specific products used at processing. This information should be recorded when the cattle arrive and provides basic data for calculating health indices, as well as information for other management and epidemiologic questions. Important rates to measure are as follows:

- *Morbidity rate*—Number of animals pulled for treatment divided by the number of animals that were received into the lot during a time period
- *Mortality rate*—Number of animals that died divided by the number of animals received during a time period[4]
- *Repeat rate*—Number of animals requiring a second treatment for the same disease occurrence divided by the total number of treatments
- *Repull rate*—Number of animals that are pulled from the pen with the same diagnosis for which they had been previously diagnosed and pulled

PEN TREATMENT CARD

Product	Date	Ser#	Location	Initials

Rework
Dates: ____________
Lot #: ____________
Wt. in: ____________

Pen #: ________
Date in: ________ #: ________

Score:
1 = Mild
2 = Moderate
3 = Severe
4 = Moribund

Date Pulled	Hosp No.	Diagnosis	Day 1				Day 2				Day 3				Date Home	Notes
			Temp	Score	Drug	Dosage	Temp	Score	Drug	Dosage	Temp	Score	Drug	Dosage		

Figure 1. Sample of a pen treatment card.

- *Chronic rate*—Number of cattle for which further treatment is deemed to be of no benefit and salvage is necessary divided by the number of cattle received during the same period

The time factor is usually defined by the user of the data and may be a month, a year, or an at risk period; alternatively, it may be useful to define the period as the time an animal spends on a production site. It is important to note that all of the indices calculated must have a time factor as part of their denominator. The denominator is not a standardized term, and care must be taken when comparing the numbers from different operations. The information gathered is used to assist in making decisions regarding large populations of animals. Frequent changes in individual animal therapies or in disease prevention programs are discouraged as this usually only serves to complicate the information and does not change the outcome. For example, the use of several different antibiotic combination therapies in the daily treatment of individual animals does little to contribute to a better understanding of appropriate therapy; however, the number of different combinations that could be evaluated requires data from large numbers of animals to sort out differences between treatments.

The responsibility of finding and removing animals from the pen due to illness or injury is generally assigned to the penchecker. The penchecker is most often a layperson who has received some training in the detection of sick animals. This task is simplified by providing a diagnostic list of common feedlot conditions to personnel involved in pulling and treating the cattle (Figure 2). This ensures some standardization of the information on the cards. The list of diagnoses must be common feedlot diseases that are familiar to personnel pulling cattle in the feedlot. If diseases or conditions are unfamiliar, training needs to be implemented.

Classifying diseases by the systems affected is a logical method of categorizing feedlot conditions. Such an organizational system seems to be easily mastered by lay personnel. The following is an outline of the classification of the important feedlot diseases.[1]

Respiratory System

- *Respiratory (pneumonia)*—This is the most common disease in feedlot cattle. Signs include anorexia, depression, nasal discharge, abnormal breathing, and a gaunt appearance. The etiology generally involves a mixed bacterial infection and may or may not have a viral component.
- *Respiratory (chronic)*—Animals with more advanced signs of respiratory infection, or animals that have been treated and have failed to respond, would fit into this classification. Signs include severe depression, rough hair coat, and a gaunt appearance. Typically, some lung pathology is associated with this classification.
- *Diphtheria*—This disease is usually an acute infection manifested by difficult, noisy breathing. The etiology can be mixed, but *Fusobacterium necrophorum* and *Haemophilus somnus* have been implicated.
- *Allergic pneumonia*—The signs are quite similar to diphtheria, except for more open mouth breathing and increased respiratory grunting sounds common in animals suffering from emphysema. Examination of the bunks may reveal some buildup of caked feed and mold. Necropsy evidence involves a heavy, wet lung that is devoid of pneumonia.
- *Honker*—This syndrome is more prevalent during hot weather and may be triggered by increased pen activity, such as when fat cattle are moved or handled and during bulling activity in a pen. The loud honking sounds made at expiration are a result of severe hemorrhage and edema of the lower tracheal mucosa-submucosa, causing obstructive dyspnea.

Digestive System

- *Bloat (ruminal tympany)*—Bloat is

System	Code Number	Diagnosis
Respiratory	1	Respiratory (pneumonia)
	2	Respiratory (chronic)
	3	Diphtheria
	4	Allergic pneumonia
	5	Honker
Digestive	6	Bloat
	7	Noneater
	8	Scours
	9	Overeating
	10	Coccidiosis
Skeletal	11	Footrot
	12	Lameness
	13	Injury
	14	Downer
Urogenital	15	OB (calving)
	16	Prolapse
	17	Uterine infection
	18	Waterbelly
Central nervous system	19	Brainer
Miscellaneous	20	Buller injury
	21	Heat stroke
	22	Unknown
	23	Miscellaneous
	24	Buller

Figure 2. Sample diagnostic list of common feedlot conditions.

caused by the inability of an animal to remove excess gas from the rumen. Bloat is either in the form of free gas or frothy bloat. It is characterized by severe distension of the rumen; when untreated, the resulting pressure on the diaphragm and thoracic cavity leads to an inability to ventilate.

■ *Non-eater*—A number of animals entering the feedlot may not readily accept the rations presented to them, they may be lower on the social pecking order, or they simply do not consume an adequate amount of feed. Therefore they seem to have a gaunt appearance when compared to other animals in their pens. Signs can be very similar to those associated with an early infection but are generally differ-

entiated by a normal respiratory rate and a normal temperature. These animals may need to be removed from their pens and placed in a less competitive feeding area.

■ *Scours*—Many digestive disorders are manifested by some type of scours or diarrhea. They may be caused by an infectious agent or simply be the result of a gastrointestinal upset due to ration change. The clinical signs of scours include the presence of loose stools in the pen, feces-smeared hindquarters, and a generally gaunt appearance of the animal.

■ *Overeating (enterotoxemia)*—Enterotoxemia is usually diagnosed at necropsy in an animal that has been on high energy ration for more than 45 days and then found dead in the pen. The signs of typical overeating include a full appearance with possible drooling, a staggering gait, and a foamy diarrhea.

- *Coccidiosis*—Bloody or a black, tarry diarrhea is generally diagnostic of coccidiosis. It occurs primarily in the first 28 days on feed. Use of preventatives is normally a routine procedure.

Musculoskeletal System

- *Footrot (infectious pododermatitis)*— The most obvious sign of footrot in feedlot cattle is lameness in one limb. Usually, swelling between the toes of the affected foot arises as a result of pathogenic invasion of this soft tissue. Differentiating this disease from BVD, founder (laminitis), or injury can be done by an examination of the involved foot. Wet conditions, sharp soil objects, and clay soils seem to provide a better environment for the agent. In addition, animals in new pens or pens that have been recently cleaned are likely to have a higher incidence of footrot.

- *Lameness*—This classification refers to animals that are obviously lame but not as a result of pododermatitis or injury (i.e., a swollen joint and/or reluctance of the animal to place weight on the limb). This type of lameness can result from a respiratory infection that has become systemic. Prognosis for affected animals is poor.

- *Injury*—Injuries to the feet and other musculoskeletal structures are not uncommon in cattle, and in many instances there is evidence of some sort of trauma. When injuries occur in greater than 1% of the cattle received, a careful inspection of facilities, handling, and transportation should be done to discover the cause.

- *Downer*—This general classification is appropriate to identify animals that are unable to rise either due to injury or chronic illness.

Urogenital System

- *Dystocia (Calving)*
- *Prolapse*—Rectal or vaginal prolapses fall under this category.
- *Uterine infection*—This commonly occurs after abortions in feedlot heifers. All heifers that have been given an abortifacient should be checked to determine if the fetus has been expelled.
- *Waterbelly*—The two main types of urinary calculi in feedlot cattle are phosphatic and silicious. Silicious calculi form from grazing grasses high in silica, and clinical signs are seen early in the feeding period. Phosphatic calculi may occur at any time in the feeding period and usually result from an imbalance in the Ca:P ratio. Ratios from 1.5:1 to 2:1 are generally recommended.

Central Nervous System

All of the central nervous system diseases are grouped under one general heading. This classification includes diseases such as polioencephalomalacia, thromboembolic meningoencephalitis, nervous coccidiosis, and brain abscesses. The signs are similar, and it is difficult for lay personnel to determine a diagnosis from the clinical signs alone. Generally, therapy is quite unrewarding except in early cases of polioencephalomalacia. A differential diagnosis based on gross and microscopic lesions is important so that prophylactic procedures can be initiated to prevent further losses.

Miscellaneous Conditions

This category includes any miscellaneous condition such as buller injury or heat stroke, as well as any unknown condition. The consulting veterinarian may need to walk or ride pens with the trainee or, more commonly, an experienced penchecker can provide the necessary training. By using information from the cards to generate the health indices, each penchecker may be evaluated. Further training or other man-

TABLE 1
Example of Management Classification System

Category	High Risk	Medium Risk	Low Risk
Morbidity (%)	30%–50% or more	20%–30%	up to 20%
Mortality (%)	2% or more	1%–2%	1% or less
Repeat treatment rate (%)	15% or more	10%–15%	10% or less
Chronic rate (%)	2% or more	1%–2%	1% or less

agement steps may be necessary to address abnormally high rates in any category. For example, a high rate of chronic respiratory disease in one pen may not be due to ineffective therapy but more often is a result of inadequate early detection of sick animals.

Accurately recording the treatments used in cases of medical intervention is vital to therapy evaluation by the veterinarian. The treatments used are ordinarily taken directly from a detailed treatment schedule provided well in advance of the arrival of cattle. The percentage of mortality, repeat treatments, repulls, chronics, and cost per head by treatment can be used to evaluate the success or failure of a particular therapy. Very high rates of success (i.e., repeat rates <5%) may indicate that too many animals are being pulled and treated unnecessarily. Treatment success rates lower than expected usually result from late detection.

Bovine Respiratory Disease

Bovine respiratory disease (BRD) accounts for 70% to 80% of all morbidity and from 30% to 60% of all mortality in beef cattle confinement feeding operations.[5,6] BRD is the most economically important disease problem that cattle feeders must overcome if they are to realize a profit.[5,6] The morbidity, mortality, and economic consequences of BRD are much higher in lightweight, high risk calves than in yearling cattle. This disease complex develops as a result of exposure of susceptible animals to respiratory pathogens at a time when the animals are undergoing stressors that decrease their ability to effectively ward off disease.

Management tools that can be used to help minimize stressors and decrease the economic impact of BRD are presented below. Although the discussion is organized under sections on prearrival, arrival, and postarrival management, many of the principles are applicable to all periods.

PREARRIVAL MANAGEMENT

History

A complete history of the animals entering a feedlot is desirable. Often this information is not available. However, some knowledge or expectation of the health performance of cattle is needed. For management purposes it is useful to divide cattle into categories or groups according to the risk of developing disease, primarily BRD. Animals are assigned to one of three risk management categories, a high risk group, a medium risk group, and a low risk group; standards for morbidity, mortality, repeat treatment rate, and chronic rate for each group are arbitrarily determined (see Table 1 for a sample). For cattle to fit into these definitions, they must fall into at least one of the expected categories, with the category with the highest rate defining the expectations. Definitions for each category or group may be changed or redefined; however, these standards should provide a starting point.

Origin

The number of pulls should also be charted as a function of days on feed (date) (Figure 3). This information can be useful in determining the timing of mass medica-

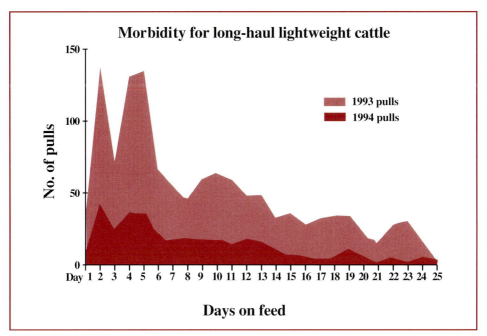

Figure 3. Number of pulls charted as a function of days on feed.

tions and/or processing procedures. Histori-cal data should include the origin of the cat-tle, with the location pinpointed as specifi-cally as possible. It is important that the environment where the cattle are fed is compatible with their needs. Customizing the handling of arrival cattle according to their specific condition (e.g., nutritional sta-tus and parasite exposure) is beneficial. For example, cattle from a selenium-deficient pasture will benefit from supplementation on arrival and demonstrate better health and performance; the additional money spent in the arrival program results in a positive return on investment.[7] The arrival program can also be customized by choosing not to administer specific products. For example, if cattle have been backgrounded in a bunk-fed environment for 90 days after receiving an anthelmintic regimen that is effective against immature and mature internal para-sites (class III dewormer), it is unlikely that another dose of anthelmintic would result in a positive return on investment. Diseases that are prevalent in the area of origin

should be taken into consideration when formulating the arrival program.

Examples of historical data that are of particular importance to the animal health program include the following:

- In lightweight calves a history of inclu-sion of cottonseed products in the ration might signal concerns regarding gossypol toxicity.[8]
- Polioencephalomalacia problems in arrival cattle might be linked to a his-tory involving corn gluten feed or turnip grazing by cattle.[9]
- When range cattle from fluke endemic areas are purchased, it is advisable to determine whether or not fluke treat-ment is needed.

Animal Health Products

It is important to learn which animal health products (i.e., specific trade names and serial numbers) the cattle received and the dates and routes by which the products were administered. With this information the veterinarian can make appropriate vaccination decisions. For example, lightweight calves that have already received two doses of vaccines against pathogens for which the feedlot normally vaccinates and that have already been implanted should probably be penned directly and not put through the chute upon arrival. Likewise, animals given a class III dewormer that have not had access to a grazing area are not likely to require another anthelmintic treatment.

Veterinary Procedures

It should be determined which veterinary procedures have been completed. For example, does a "load of steers" contain all castrated males or are some of the males still intact? In addition to the obvious adjustment in the value of the animals, the use of *Clostridium tetani* products would be considered if the feedyard bands bulls. A similar pertinent piece of information about heifers would be their pregnancy/spay status. Depending on the exposure risk, commingling of cattle at the time of purchase, and palpation of a test population, the decision is made whether or not to test for pregnancy and abort as needed. In the case of spayed heifers, money can be saved by not performing pregnancy tests and also by deleting melengestrol acetate (MGA) from the ration.

Nutritional Status

The importance of the historical nutritional information on new cattle is often underestimated or ignored totally. Nutritional status not only refers to feedstuffs that the calves have been eating but also information about whether the cattle are weaned and are trained to eat from a bunk and drink from a water tank. It may also include details about body condition and hair as they relate to dietary exposure to micronutrient or fungal toxins.

Cattle that come to the feedlot lacking an acceptable balance of micronutrients may have health problems. Inadequate levels of vitamin A,[10] vitamin E,[10] beta-carotene,[10] selenium,[10] copper,[11] and zinc[11] have been associated with poor immune

response upon feedlot arrival. Low vitamin A levels decrease the humoral immune response in ruminants,[12] whereas animals given selenium supplementation are more resistant to clinical infections. In a study involving lambs challenged with parainfluenza virus, Reffett and coworkers[13] demonstrated that vitamin E and selenium improved immune response independent of each other.[14] Cattle previously exposed to mycotoxins of moldy feed may arrive at the feedlot with impaired immune function[15]; thus these animals will be unable to properly respond to a vaccination program.

Transportation
Transit Time

The amount of time that calves spend away from a home pen environment is the transit time (from the time the calves leave home until they arrive at the feedlot). In the case of auction markets, this is more than the trucking time. This period represents a physiologically stressful times for these animals; as a result, the circulating glucocorticoid level increases[16] and is accompanied by dehydration, making affected animals more susceptible to disease.[17,18] Every effort should be made to minimize transit time. Animals should be allowed free access to water and a high quality roughage-based ration prior to shipping. The goal is to have the ration provide adequate energy and protein levels to maintain rumen function throughout the trip.

Quality Transit

Trucking firms generally have made significant improvement in their willingness to help keep cattle healthy while in their care. Recommendations to help maximize the effectiveness of the cattle truckers in these efforts include the following:

- Make sure that the exhaust system is functioning properly and does not have leaks that could be sucked into the trailer and that the exhaust pipe is long enough to keep truck exhaust out of the trailer. If there is an exhaust problem, it can be detected inside the trailer as soon as the truck stops (often the odor can be noticed by smelling the hair of the cattle). Truck exhaust can impair the mucociliary blanket involved in dust and pathogen clearance. Disrupting this system leads to invasion of deeper tissues in the respiratory tract and, ultimately, to pneumonia.[19]

- Minimize the use of electric shock prods. In addition to increasing the likeness of bruising the animals, excessive use of a prod on abrasive floor surfaces increases the animals' risk of developing rear toe abrasions, which lead to non–weight-bearing lameness, poor performance, and, occasionally, complications requiring euthanasia.
- Trucks should be cleaned prior to collecting a load of calves to decrease the risk of exposure to pathogens from previous cattle.
- Avoid overcrowding on the truck.
- Check cattle every 2 hours to make sure that all cattle are standing.

Facility Checklist

The facility that is used to work and hold cattle also has an impact on how well cattle start on feed, the rate of BRD in these cattle, and how well they respond to therapy if they develop BRD.

Arrival Pen

Prior to calf arrival, the arrival area should be inspected (if not already done so on a regular basis by an assigned person). In the arrival pens the fence must be in good repair and should be readily visible and sturdy. If the feed bunk serves as part of the pen perimeter, the neck bar or cables should be adjusted appropriately for the size of cattle coming to the pen. The arrival period is the time during the feeding period when cattle are most likely to escape from their pens. If the feedlot has pens designated for arrival only, the tanks are best placed along the perimeter fences, so the cattle will encounter them while walking around the perimeter of the pen; this is especially

important for weaning calves. Tanks should be cleaned. If possible, raise the water level in the tank so that the basin is full, making it easier for the cattle to find the water. Depending on the origin of the cattle, consider adding a small hose running into the tank so that the cattle can hear and see the running water, as this may help cattle that have only been stream drinkers and are not tank-broke. If the pens are dirt pens, they should be in good repair, with no mud or erosion barriers to the tank or bunk pad. There should be no standing water in the pens, since cattle will generally drink the first water that they come to without respect for flavor or infectious potential.

Processing Area

Physical injuries and cuts leading to lameness can be the stressors that keep cattle away from the tank and bunk, hence putting them at risk of developing BRD. Part of the arrival facility assessment includes walking through the entire facility after it has been cleaned to look for sharp corners, loose or worn metal, and any areas that might cause cuts or bruises. Make certain that the facility is in good repair and operational before filling it with cattle. Careful, quiet handling of cattle through the sorting pens, tub, circle, and chute is of foremost importance. Prior to cattle arrival, compare the processing program with the equipment available. It is advisable to have at least one backup piece of equipment for each procedure being performed. Equipment should be checked to ensure that it is operational and properly calibrated so that the proper dosages of products are administered. Review the cleaning and operational procedures to ensure that modified live vaccines are not at risk of being inactivated by disinfectants.

ARRIVAL MANAGEMENT

Cattle Assessment
Quality as Represented

Cattle quality is usually a function of genetics and nutrition and therefore is not directly linked to BRD. However, if on arrival the cattle appear to be significantly different than represented, the history presented with the cattle should be reevaluated. If the decision is made to keep the cattle, a more conservative processing program for the cattle may be needed.

Health as Represented

Cattle that are represented as ranch-fresh bawling calves with a short haul should not have a gaunt, stale look. They should be expected to be clean, slick-haired calves with at least average fill. Special attention should be given to calves with excessive shrink for their transit time or calves transported through adverse weather conditions.

Processing Programs

The specific combination of vaccines, implants, and parasiticide products used on cattle coming into the feedlot vary with class of cattle, region, season, and recommendation of the veterinarian. Any attempt to discuss all possible combinations would be cumbersome and of limited use. Instead, this discussion will center around the major classes of products commonly used. Please note that with many of the products, there are often several manufacturers with similar label claims.

Respiratory Viral Vaccine

Respiratory viral vaccines represent the major class of vaccines that are used in the feedlot industry to protect against morbidity, mortality, and economic losses. The four most common viral antigens included are infectious bovine rhinotracheitis (IBR), parainfluenza 3 virus (PI$_3$), bovine viral diarrhea (BVD) virus, and bovine respiratory syncytial virus (BRSV). The virus vaccines are available as killed, modified live, and combinations of killed and modified live products. Injectable products stimulate the immune system by causing an increase in humoral (IgG and IgM circulating antibody)[20] and cell-mediated immunity (modified live products).[20] In addition to the traditional injectable vaccines, modified live intranasal products that contain IBR and PI$_3$ are also available. These products have a mode of action that causes increased surface immunity (IgA) and nonspecific immunity through the mediation of interferon.[20]

Respiratory Bacterial Vaccine

Bacterial vaccination to protect animals from the clinical disease caused by *Pasteurella haemolytica, Pasteurella multocida,* and *Haemophilus somnus* is used, primarily in lightweight calves. Vaccine can be whole cell bacterins or the more efficacious products containing somatic antigens as well as a toxoid fraction. With the toxoid technology, products offer humoral antibody protection against bacterial cell colonization, as well as neutralization of the leukotoxin produced by the bacterial cell.[20] Also available are nonspecific vaccinations that provide for the development of humoral antibodies directed against the J chain fragment of the endotoxin produced during gram-negative infections.

Mass Medication Considerations

Normally, the decision to administer mass medication to arrival cattle is based on the history, origin, season, and previous experience in the feedlot. Thus the decision is usually made in the prearrival phase. On the occasion that the feedlot receives cattle that are higher risk than expected or ones that had extraordinary stress during the trucking phase, the decision to mass medicate or refuse to take delivery of the cattle must be made as the animals exit the truck.

Mass medication of arrival cattle to reduce the likelihood of BRD should be considered in cases of high risk calves in which we expect to have high and early morbidity from bacterial or viral pneumonia. The route of administration and product selection should be based on origin of the cattle and severity of anticipated disease.

Feed Antimicrobials. Feeding antimicrobials to calves in the early postarrival period can help increase feed intake[21,22] and average daily gain and decrease morbidity and mortality rates.[22] Tetracycline or tetracycline-sulfa drug combinations have been used for over 25 years for prevention and control of BRD.[22] Feed additive products are generally used over extended periods for animals that are healthy on arrival.

Water-Soluble Products. Water-soluble antimicrobial products can be effective when given to new arrivals into the feedlot. Cattle consume water as they are unloaded from the truck in linear proportion to their percentage shrink and with little regard to the flavor of the water. It should be noted that cattle may consume considerably less than 1 gal/cwt/day, as commonly suggested.[23] Data generated at various times of the year on various classes of cattle indicate that the daily intakes are more often in the range of 0.5 gal/cwt/day. The effect of water-soluble products on rumen fermentation is negligible as evidenced by rumen volatile fatty acids produced.[23] Water-soluble products should be considered when arrival cattle are coming to the feedlot at a time when water systems are not in danger of freezing and when high morbidity is expected within the first few days following arrival of cattle.

Injectables. High risk cattle that come to the feedyard and that have been subject to excessive commingling, disease exposure, and high stress are candidates for injectable mass medication. The usefulness of injectable mass medication, like that of water-soluble products, is greatest in animals that will likely experience BRD within the first week of placement in the feedlot; these products would not be expected to have a significant effect in situations where the animals have had a chance to respond to an effective vaccination program.

Managing the Feed Bunk. It is important to pay special attention to ration and bunk management during the arrival period. By nature, most cattle that are coming to the feedlot from a pasture situation will avoid the concentrate portions of the ration. Often, the calves tend to sort the feed and eat only the long stem hay for a few days. The challenge is to provide adequate levels of energy, protein, and micronutrients to these calves. Nutrient formulation suggestions are not covered in detail in this discussion. However, it is important to note that rations must be sufficiently enriched with micronutrients to account for the low percent of body weight intake that the animals are actually consuming; we must also recognize that using the average daily intake for a pen does not account for the most "at risk animals," which are the ones that have a low intake. Rations for newly arrived calves should not contain fermented feeds initially, they should be palatable, and they should not be too dry or powdery, as this decreases palatability.

Adequate pen and bunk space helps to minimize stress on the animals. Calves should have at least 12 inches of bunk space and 25 square feet of pen space. In concrete arrival pens a space of 100 square feet per animal[24] is acceptable for short periods.

POSTARRIVAL MANAGEMENT

Management of cattle after they have been placed in their home pens is critical in the occurrence, recognition, and treatment of BRD cases.

Recognition of BRD

Early recognition, early treatment, and early return to the home pen environment are the most important criteria to consider when evaluating response to therapy. Calves with BRD are lethargic and dyspneic. They often stand or lie off by themselves (easily noted when the other calves are at the bunk), and they commonly have rectal temperatures in excess of 104.0° F. The animal may appear to be gaunt, although not necessarily very early in the disease process.

Hospital Management

The purpose of a hospital facility within a feedlot is to provide a place for animals to recover from an injury or infection in a low stress, low competition environment that provides easy access to fresh water and fresh fortified rations and a comfortable place to rest under the watchful eye of a hospital manager. The role of the hospital manager is to provide the aforementioned properties, evaluate the individual animal's response to therapy, and be willing to reevaluate the initial diagnosis and to change therapeutic regimens, if necessary.

Minimizing Stress

A large portion of BRD prevention in the postarrival period can be grouped under the broad category of stress-minimizing activities. Managing the rations and bunks relative to weather changes can help minimize the stress associated with acidosis, thus decreasing the BRD commonly seen after acidosis outbreaks. Pen maintenance to help control dust and minimize lameness problems can also help minimize stressors.

SUMMARY

Health programs based solely on vaccination and treatment regimens are often short lived and unrewarding. The basis of any successful ongoing health program is a working health management system. The key to the success of any system is a functioning record system that generates information that is meaningful to management. The basic information generated should be the incidence of morbidity and mortality, as well as the number of repeat treatments, repulls, and chronic calves. A goal or expectation for these measurements for different categories of cattle based on weight, age, nutritional status, and distance hauled should be in place. If goals are not reached, reasons can be investigated. The most common reason for expectations not being achieved is due to factors that are largely beyond the control of the feedyard. While attempts to address these factors should be made, the focus of the health program should be on the factors that are controllable at the feedyard. Each component of

the health program needs to be evaluated, and the changes should be made as required to address specific problems.

Bovine respiratory disease is the most important economic disease in the feedlot. Prearrival management is extremely important in assessing the risk category of incoming calves and in applying various preventive health strategies. Knowledge of the origin, background, and previous preventive health measures of cattle is very useful information and assists in the determination of measures needed upon their arrival at the feedlot. In addition, good husbandry practice and proper nutrition help to minimize the stressful conditions that accompany large feeding operations.

REFERENCES

1. Edwards AJ, Stokka GL: Feedlot health management, in Howard J (ed): *Current Veterinary Therapy 2: Food Animal Practice.* Philadelphia, WB Saunders, 1986, pp 135–142.
2. Bebbet RM: Case study of a simple decision support system to aid livestock disease control decisions. *Agri Syst* 38:111–129, 1992.
3. Weaver LD, Payne MA, Wong WS, Murray WM: Use of computerized food animal medical records for disease surveillance and residue avoidance. *Compend Contin Educ Pract Vet* 14(7):981–985, 1992.
4. Smith RD: *Veterinary Clinical Epidemiology.* Stoneman, MA, Butterworth Heinemann, 1991.
5. Vogel GJ, Parrott C: Mortality survey in feedlots: The incidence of death from digestive, respiratory, and other death losses. *Scientific Update on Rumensin/Tylan for the Professional Feedlot Consultant.* Canyon, TX, Elanco Animal Health/Lilly Research Laboratories, 1993, p 21.
6. USDA, National Agriculture Statistical Service, Cattle and Calves Death Loss, May 1992.
7. Lechtenberg KF: Unpublished data, Rhea Cattle Co., 1988–1994.
8. Holmberg C: Pathology related to gossypol toxicity in calves. Proceedings of the Academy of Veterinary Consultants, Dec 1990.
9. Wilkse SE, Leathers CW, Parish SM: Diseases of cattle that graze turnips. *Comp Food Anim* 9(3):113–121, 1987.
10. Nockels CF: Micronutrients and the immune response. *Vet Med,* Winter/Spring 1991, pp 14–17.
11. Niederman CN, Blodgett D, Eversole D, et al: Effect of copper and iron on neutrophil function and humoral immunity of gestating beef cattle. *JAVMA* 204(11):1796–1800, 1994.

12. Bruns NJ, Webb Jr KE: Vitamin A deficiency: Serum cortisol and humoral immunity in lambs. *J Anim Sci* 68:454–459, 1990.

13. Reffett JK, Spears JW, Brown TT Jr: Effect of dietary selenium and vitamin E on the primary and secondary immune response in lambs challenged with parainfluenza virus. *J Anim Sci* 66:1520–1528, 1988.

14. Erskine RJ, Eberhart RJ, Grasso PJ, Scholz RW: Induction of *Escherichia coli* mastitis in cows fed selenium-deficient or selenium-supplemented diets. *Am J Vet Res* 50(12):2093–2100, 1989.

15. Osweiler GD: Mycotoxins and livestock: What role do fungal toxins play in illness and production losses? *Vet Med* 85(1):89–94, 1990.

16. Agnes F, Sartorelli P, Abdi BH, Locatelli A: Effect of transport loading or noise on blood biochemical variables in calves. *Am J Vet Res* 51(10):1679–1681, 1990.

17. Breazile JE: The physiology of stress and its relationship to mechanisms of disease and therapeutics. *Vet Clin North Am Food Anim Pract* 4(3):441–480, 1988.

18. Sconberg S, Nockels CF, Bennett BW, et al: Effects of shipping, handling, adrenocorticotropic hormone, and epinephrine on alpha-tocopherol content of bovine blood. *Am J Vet Res* 54(8):1287–1293, 1993.

19. Vestwebber JG: Diseases of the respiratory system, in Howard J (ed): *Current Veterinary Therapy 2: Food Animal Practice*. Philadelphia, WB Saunders, 1986, pp 657–666.

20. Roth J: Vaccination-Immunology, influencing factors and interactions, in *Biologicals, Vaccination, and Immunity*. Academy of Veterinary Consultants, Aurora, CO, Dec 5–7, 1991, Vol XIX, No 3, pp 1–26. Courtesy of Microbial Genetics, a Division of Pioneer Hi-Bred-International Inc.

21. Hawley GE: Control of the shipping fever complex with terramycin in feedlot rations. *Vet Med,* October 1957, pp 481–484.

22. Technical bulletin 25, American Cyanamid, Auero S 700, Medicated PreMix.

23. Lechtenberg KF: Factors affecting water consumption in feedlot cattle, in *Parasite Control, Water Consumption, Veterinarians and Nutritionists, Acute Phase Proteins and Salmonellosis*. Academy of Veterinary Consultants, Amarillo, TX, Jun 3–5, 1993, pp 16–26.

24. Guidelines for beef cattle husbandry, in *Guide for the Care and Use of Agricultural Research and Teaching,* ed 1. Mar 1988, pp 23–27.